# The Medical Key
# to the Doctrine of the Chinese
# on Pulses

## Michal Boym

## English Edition

## Translated by
## Shawn Daniels, Ph.D

The Medical Key to the Doctrine of the Chinese on Pulses
Michal Boym
English Edition
Translated by Shawn Daniels, Ph.D

Soul Care Publishing
Vancouver, Canada
SoulCarePublishing.com

# Table of Contents

# About the Translator

Shawn Daniels, Ph.D.

Shawn Daniels received his PhD in Classical Humanities from the University of Florida in 2013, focusing on Latin literature in late antiquity. Aside from being a translator, he is also an adjunct professor at Wright State University and the online Latin teacher for the Beachwood school district in Cleveland, Ohio.

# Foreword

It is with great pleasure that I was asked to write a foreword for this new translation of Michał Boym's *"Clavis Medica ad Chinarum doctrinam de pulsibus"* (The Medical Key to the Chinese Doctrines of the Pulse), translated by Shawn Daniels, Ph.D. Although Boym research has always been a key topic for Sinology, Chinese President's Xi Jin-ping's quotations on the People's Daily about the significant contributions of the Polish missionary in introducing China to the west facilitated his induction into the pantheon of the state approved "Belt and Road Initiative" pre-modern visionaries. In this sense, this book is not only an important achievement for Sinology, but also makes a strong statement about current world affairs.

## A. The life of Michał Boym

The life of Michał Boym (1612-1659) has been explored in detail, in the famous article by Paul Pelliot[1]. Several mistakes in Pelliot's work were rectified mainly through the works of Prof. Boleslaw Szczesniak, Edward Kajdański, Noël Golvers and several others who meticulously examined and studied Boym's legacy. For this reason it is very difficult to produce a similarly original recount of Boym's life without copying the information already written by them.

Therefore, this is a short summary of his life, which may allow the reader to understand his background, his trips to Asia and his momentous contributions to Sinology.

Paweł Jerzy Boim (1581–1641, Michał's father was an imperial Physician, and therefore, according to the practices of the era, Michał Boym was predestined to carry forward his father's legacy. Boym however did not become a doctor, but joined the Catholic Church. Being a member of the high society and associating with people of the letters, Boym received not only a good medical training and also a full classical education, becoming very well versed in Latin and Greek. In

---

[1] Paul Pelliot. Michel Boym. T'oung Pao, Volume 31, Issue 1. 1934. pages 95 – 151

essence Boym was a prominent scholar even prior to his trips to China. In 1643 he left Europe and traveled to the Far East, where he journeyed around Vietnam and China. In Macau he arrived in 1650, and became a Professor at St. Joseph's College[2]. However, within the same year he embarked on an ambassadorial work at the to the court of the Ming pretender Yongli (永曆帝), to support Fr. Andreas Wolfgang Koffler (1612- 1652)[3], and departed from Macau on January 1st 1651. After 1651, Boym never returned to Macau again.

After arriving in Guangxi he acted as a liaison between the Pope and the Southern Ming Court. He was eventually sent to Rome to deliver letters from the newly converted empress dowager Helena to the Pope Innocent X, which were requesting for assistance against the Qing (i.e. the Manchu). In 1651 Boym started his journey back to Rome, finally reaching the "Eternal City" in 1652. Unfortunately, Boym's support for the Ming was largely unpopular, and travelling to Rome was seen as a dangerous move that could endanger the China mission. Upon arrival the Vatican was reluctant to side with either side and in the meantime a change of Pope further delayed response. Finally Boym met with Pope Alexander VII in the December of 1655, almost three years after arriving in Rome.

Pope Alexander provided him with letters of support for the Yongli pretender, and appointed him leader of a team of faithful companions, which included Philippe Couplet. Couplet would later inherit the bulk of Boym's medical manuscripts prior to their publication in Europe. However, in 1658, while still en route, Boym was ordered not to return to Macau because the Portuguese had already gained the support of the Qing court. Therefore he changed his traveling arrangements and finally arrived in Guangxi by pirate ship in 1659, where he died from exhaustion soon after. It is not clear if the Papal letters ever reached the Yongli pretender's Court.

---

[2] Vide Krzyszkowski, Michał Boym, S.J., Misje Katolickie, Krakow, 1929, 48:307-327.

[3] Claudia Von Collani. A missionary on his journey: Michał Boym and Religions in East Asia. Monumenta Serica Vol. 59 , Iss. 1,2011

Michal Boym

## B. Boym's Linguistics in China Illustrata and published works in Rome

The discovery of the Nestorian Stele was one of the most important discoveries of the Jesuits. At the time, the discovery did not hold an archaeological as much as a religious significance. The Jesuits believed that if Eastern Christianity was able to break the cultural barriers that the Jesuits could not, there was hope for the future.

Boym apparently never personally visited the stele[4] but accessed its text from a book by E. Diaz named "T'ang Ching-chiao pei-sung cheng-ch'uan" 《唐景教碑頌正詮》 published in Wu-Lin Hangchow in the year 1644[5].

Being naturally curious about this early Christian text, he copied the characters, and provided a phonetic transliteration in Cantonese. In addition he included a Latin translation for every character on that list. The deciphering of the Nestorian Stele by Boym was officially the first list of word correspondences between Chinese and Latin. As such, Boym's list, which was first published by Kircher, can be perceived as the earliest Sino-European dictionary, and the beginning of Chinese lexicography. Additionally to this, Kircher and others[6] subscribed to a theory that linked Chinese characters to Egyptian Hieroglyphics. Boym being fascinated by the Chinese characters, he worked on a project that would explain the development of the Hanzi as a representation of hidden ideas behind the strokes. His conclusions offer a remarkable view of how he tried to break down the hidden linguistic codes of the ancient Chinese and make sense of the

---

[4] Feza Günergun, Dhruv RainaScience between Europe and Asia: Historical Studies on the Transmission, Adoption and Adaptation of Knowledge.Springer Science & Business Media, 2010 p 217
[5] Boleslaw Szcześniak and Michael Boym. The Beginnings of Chinese Lexicography in Europe with Particular Reference to the Work of Michael Boym (1612-1659). Journal of the American Oriental Society, Vol. 67, No. 3 (Jul. - Sep., 1947), pp. 160- 165
[6] Boleslaw Szczesniak. The Origin of the Chinese Language According to Athanasius Kircher's Theory. Journal of the American Oriental Society, Vol. 72, No. 1 (Jan. - Mar., 1952), pp. 21-29

pictograms. However his work is now severely outdated, especially since the discovery of the Oracle Bones (甲骨文), which allowed us to understand the development of the Chinese characters from their earliest form down to modern versions much more clearly and scientifically.

Boym's linguistic capabilities are vital for understanding his writings, because prior to his work there were no Medical Dictionaries or Glossaries of any kind to assist with translation. Boym had to personally invent a terminology, a translation theory, and the practical methods to convey the Chinese ideas into Latin words.

In the Vatican Library also exist various maps drawn by Boym[7]. It appears that Boym and the Jesuit Mission in Macau were very interested in knowing the terrain, and the specific geographic conditions of China[89]. Boym's hand-drawn maps offered a first look of the various Chinese provinces, and were invaluable for the Vatican. The accuracy and trivialities of those maps are not the focus of this paper, but the fact that such documents exist reveals the diversity and range of subjects that Boym investigated while in China.

While Boym was waiting for three years in Rome, he also published a number of books, the most important of which being the "Flora Sinensis" 1656[10]. "Flora Sinensis" was one of the earliest natural history books, detailing information about the various plants and the animals of the Chinese continent, and it exerted much interest and influence for the development of Zoology and Botany in Europe.

---

[7] Chinese Books and Documents in the Jesuit Archives in Rome. A Descriptive Catalogue. Japonica- Sinica I-IV by Robert Wardy. Monumenta Serica, Vol. 50 (2002), pp. 463-480

[8] Boleslaw Szczesniak (1965) The Mappa Imperii Sinarum of Michael Boym, Imago Mundi, 19:1, 113-115,

[9] Boleslaw Szczesniak. The Atlas and Geographic Description of China: A Manuscript of Michael Boym (1612-1659). Journal of the American Oriental Society, Vol. 73, No. 2 (Apr. - Jun., 1953), pp. 65-77

[10] Michał Piotr Boym. Flora Sinensis. Typis Matthaei Rictij, Viennae 1656

Michal Boym

Posthumously, Boym has been associated more with the Chinese medical works that he compiled during his stay in Macau, in Rome and in Guangxi, yet his greatest contributions are perhaps towards the field of Sinology, where his works are still quite relevant.

## C. Scholars often associated with Boym's medical publications

1. Philippe Couplet

Philippe Couplet (1623-1692) was Boym's companion on his return trip to China from Rome, and inherited and edited his writings. According to Golvers[11], he appears to have authored at least the first part of Boym's "Specimen". His correspondence with Andreas Cleyer was pivotal for the salvaging; transporting and publishing Boym's medical books in Europe.

2. Andreas Cleyer

Andreas Cleyer (1634 – c.1698) was a German doctor, based in Batavia (present day Jakarta) and he is typically regarded as the editor of Boym's published medical works (i.e. The Specimen and the Clavis). Among the scholars who study Boym's works, he is often regarded as a controversial scholar, and a plagiarist[12][13]. After Boym's books reached his hands, he tried to claim ownership. The extent of his plagiarism is very difficult to be estimated.

## D. The book that you're holding in your hands

The book that you're holding in your hands is a new translation for Boym's *"Clavis Medica ad Chinarum doctrinam de pulsibus"* (The

---

[11] Noël Golvers. Philippe Couplet, S.J. (1623–1693) and the authorship of Specimen "Medicinae Sinensis" and some other Western writings on Chinese medicine. Medizinhistorisches Journal, Bd. 35, H. 2 (2000), pp. 175-182

[12] Boleslaw Szczesniak. John Floyer and Chinese Medicine. Osiris, Vol. 11 (1954), pp. 156

[13] Edward Kajdański. Michael Boym's "Medicus Sinicus". T'oung Pao, Second Series, Vol. 73, Livr. 4/5 (1987), pp. 166

Medical Key to the Chinese doctrines of the pulse). Andreas Cleyer, under unclear circumstances published this volume in Nuremberg, in 1686. Although several pulse manuscripts are attributed to Boym, the *Clavis* is the only one that Cleyer did not claim for himself. Unfortunately for Boym, his manuscripts were printed after the publication of Harvey's circulation experiment. The shift in epistemology in the second half of the 17th century, allowed medical doctors to start moving away from empirical ancient and classical pulse theories, and eventually adopt medical practices verified through the experimental method.

## E. Boym's understanding of Chinese Medicine

Since the China Mission was manned by some of the most brilliant Jesuits scholars of the era, Boym was handpicked for his outstanding education and capabilities. His work, genius, talents and skills are undisputed, and his published work remains a testament to the origins of Sinology.

However, Boym officially lived in South East Asia from 1643 to 1650, and also for an unspecified time (perhaps several weeks) prior to his death. During that time he traveled much between Vietnam and China, without staying for lengthy periods of times in one place.

His works include monographs and notes in such diverse fields including geography, cartography, linguistics, religion, philology, astronomy, mathematics, zoology, botany and medicine. Having pursued so many areas of knowledge it is quite debatable of how many of those fields he actually mastered during his short lifetime. Having such a wide range of interests, it's apparent that Boym's focus was not always medicine.

Also, it is quite questionable how well Boym understood Chinese medicine. The study of a traditional medical system, requires complete dedication over several years, which Boym obviously can't claim.

Realistically speaking, it is very unlikely that Boym had the knowledge and experience required to translate a Chinese Medicine Corpus on his own. Therefore, given the amount of medical works

Michal Boym

(published or otherwise) associated with his name, it is very likely that many portions of his books were produced through a collective effort of the Jesuits in South East Asia.

Yet accepting that Michał Boym had a pivotal role in procuring and editing such a remarkable collection of translated works on Chinese Medicine, it's nothing sort of a feat for early Sinology.

## F. Boym's books and authorship

In China the current academic interest in Boym's work comes from the publication of a volume entitled *"International Chinese Culture Research Library: Boym's Collective Works – Chinese and Western Cultural Exchanges and Medical Correspondences"* [11] anthologized by the famous Sinologist Edward Kajdański, and translated into Chinese by Zhang Zhen-hui (张振辉) and Zhang Xi-ping (张西平) in 2013.

This book translated Boym's *"Clavis"*, *"Specimen"*, *"Flora Sinensis"* and other essays into mandarin, allowing the Chinese Medical scholars to study Boym's works for the first time in a language that they can understand.

The medical works of Michał Boym that specifically contain information about Chinese pulse diagnosis are mainly collected in two volumes. The first is the *"Specimen medicinae sinicae, sive Opuscula medica ad mentem Sinensium"* (Chinese Medicine works, or Medical Essays according to the Chinese thought), which was published in Frankfurt in 1682. The second one is this book that you're holding in your hands, i.e. the *"Clavis Medica ad Chinarum doctrinam de pulsibus"* (The Medical Key to the Chinese doctrines of the pulse) published in 1686 in Nürnberg, again by Andreas Cleyer (Andreas Cleyerus) and Philippe Couplet (Philippo Copletio). In addition, the "Clavis" was contained as an appendix to the fourth volume of the periodical: *"Miscellanea Curiosa Sive Ephemeridum Medico-Physicarum Germanicarum Academiae Naturae Curiosorum Decuriae"* [7], which was also printed in 1686.

Arguments pertaining to the authorship and other adventures of the *"Specimen"* and the *"Clavis"* have been the focus of academic disputes lasting for centuries. However although alternative opinions may still linger in academic circles, Boym's authorship, translation and editing of -at least part of- these works[8] is undeniable.

Copies of the *"Clavis"* and the *"Specimen"* are held at important European Libraries such as the National Library of France, The Bavarian State Library, The National Library of the Czech Republic and The Austrian National Library, and they have recently become available in an electronic form via relevant websites.

Besides the "Clavis" important pulse essays are also contained in the *"Specimen"*. This is evident from its list of contents:

I.      *De pulsibus libros quatuor è sinico translatos.*
II.     *Tractatus de pulsibus ab erudito europaeo collectos.*
III.    *Fragmentum operis medici ibidem ab erudito europaeo conscripti.*
IV.     *Excerpta literis eruditi europaei in China.*
V.      *Schemata ad meliorem praecedentium intelligentiam.*
VI.     *De indiciis morborum ex linguae coloribus & affectionibus (cum figuris aeneis & ligneis).*

Relevant to pulse information located in the "Specimen", Kajdański[10] mentions alternative prints of the *"De indiciis morborum ex linguae coloribus & affectionibus"*, *"Herbarium parvum"* and *"Tractatus de pulsibus"* dated 1681, that may have been published and sold by a certain August Vindel in separate brochures. I am not aware if Kajdański was ever able to locate a copy of these prints, or where they may be found.

Michal Boym

According to Kajdański again, the *Fragmentum operis medici ibidem ab erudito europaeo conscripti* may have been the last four chapters of the *Clavis*, although it was not printed as such[14].

Other pulse essays contained in the *Excerpta literis eruditi europaei in China* do not belong to Boym since their dates suggest to have been compiled many years after Boym's passing.

## G. Overdue Research on the Clavis and the Specimen

This book that you're holding in your hands still holds many secrets. Boym's work has been much distorted and sadly only printed in fragments due to the historical circumstances mentioned above. Yet, even after so many centuries there has never been a complete attempt to put together all the fragments and conclusively attach each piece of the puzzle to a specific Chinese text. Names of authors such as Huang Di and Wang Shu-he or books such as the Mai Jing and Mai Jue get mentioned often in the print text. Now that Chinese literacy is not a rare specialty anymore, translations of many classic Chinese pulse books have become popular in the west, and previously rare Chinese texts are also widely available in print or electronically, this task is much more feasible than ever before in history. This book is therefore a pivotal attempt towards that direction. I think that the modern Chinese Medicine reader or those involved in the fields of Humanities, Medical Anthropology or Sinology will greatly benefit from such an investigation and gain much perspective about Boym's impact within their own respective fields. This book is a vital step towards finally and decisively understanding and appreciating Boym's work in context that has been missing from bibliography until now.

Ioannis Solos Phd
Doctor of Medicine, Chinese Medical Author, Sinologist
Guangzhou, China 20/7/2018

---

[14] Edward Kajdański. Michael Boym's "Medicus Sinicus". T'oung Pao, Second Series, Vol. 73, Livr. 4/5 (1987), pp. 172

Medical Key to the Doctrine of the Chinese on Pulses

Michal Boym

# The Medical Key
## To the Doctrine of the Chinese
## On Pulses

By Reverend Father Michael Boymo,
from the Society Of Jesus, and a missionary in China.

Fragments of this work, buried for over twenty years and distributed all over, have been collected and published in Europe, in thanks to the Faculty of Medicine, by The Renowned Master Andreas Cleyer, Medical Doctor and Chief Physician of the Dutch East India Company[15] who has now at last sent *A Sample of the Entire Work, Recently brought from China and cleansed of mistakes* with the sponsorship of The Reverend Father Philip Coplet, The Belgian, from the Society of Jesus, Sent to Rome for a mission to China.

--------------------

In the year 1686

---

[15] *M.D. & Societatis Batavo-Orientalis Proto-Medicus*

# To the Creator Of Life and Salvation, the Prince Supreme of Physicians, Christ Jesus

To whom would I rather dedicate and consecrate this work than to You, the Creator of life and the Redeemer? Whether I deem this work as something that might give[16] remarkable fame to that workshop of the human body, certainly it should be dedicated to you in particular, who are the architect of so marvelous a workshop. If I ponder the most beautiful agreement and harmony of our small bodies, and of our human lives, alongside the enormous circuit of the heavens and every device, I should worship you chiefly! I should worship you only! You who distribute all things in their weight and measure, up until the very end, so sure and fine, even in the least of things, too; you are a great God! But if I bend my eyes toward the abundance of rivers and streams of the world, its veins, I say, and slenderest passages, through which life itself is carried and shared itself, all coming from a single spring, I would be quite the knave if I allowed them to trace this spring to anyone else than you, who are the Alpha and the Omega,[17] the beginning, I say, and the end; to any other, I say, than, as to you, the ocean of all good things, to whom all of creation courses, like rivers to the sea; but if they go astray, it is necessary that it is immediately dried out and entirely fails. To whom else, I say, than, as to you, who are the eternal Wisdom, spying our kidneys and hearts, as you can, and thus wish all to be saved!

You had made man immortal, you had also planted a tree of life; but (alas!), harmful to God and to himself, he polluted himself and all his offspring with the lethal poison of his sin, until at last, taking pity on us, you came down from heaven, the great

---

[16] *...hoc opus considero ut notitiam dare...* "I consider this work as to give fame," a strange construction. I suspect it's modeling itself after Greek natural result clauses, which suggest something is likely to follow the premise, but not absolutely.

[17] *qui es α. & ω.*

Michal Boym

Doctor—indeed, you even wanted to be called the Doctor, to be honored forever because of that necessity, unavoidable and entirely untreatable if your almighty hand had not bestowed a cure. Indeed, for you to have cast out the diseases of the soul, which are a forecast of eternal death, your divine Wisdom hardly used any other way or means more effective than tending to bodies. So you went, through the Castles and Cities, by curing all of their ailments; indeed, you deigned to apply certain medicines, made from mud or spit or waters, such that you brought everyone to recognition of You and the eternal Father by healing them of their souls' wounds. Indeed, to show that you were the true Doctor, you wanted to bear our ailments and afflictions yourself, and to carry our sorrows; that we would be cleansed by Your wound, you gave us Your body, I say, and Your blood for a cure; You were willing to die that we might live; to suffer evil, that we might enjoy good. Take also the tally of our lives, which you had made saved, to our great fortune! Not content with this, but You even left medicines for the soul, like healthful springs—that is, You left the Sacraments for a cure, among which are the sanctified body and blood, a supremely divine and life-giving cure-all, by which you tend to your own sheep with your own blood.

Therefore, this Key to You! To you, who alone open and close; to you, who have revealed, to us and to Your faith, China, which has been hidden for so many centuries.

I expect no other pay for my efforts, except for you to make the blind open their eyes, and the deaf their ears, and make the tongues of the mute speak fluently, that your praises may ring with them forever, and last, that they might recognize your Father, and You the Son, whom the Father sent, Jesus Christ; for this is eternal life, that we may be brought out of this universal hospital[18] of our exile into eternal blessedness, and cross in time,

[18] Going back to the Greek original, νοσοκομεῖον, it could also mean "bed-chamber;" maybe something like "waiting room"?

with the lines of the Chinese joined, to the Land that knows no illness and death.

Michael Boymus, Society of Jesus.

Michal Boym

Reverend Father Michael Boymus

Of the Society of Jesus, from the Kingdom of Siam

# Preface to the Reader

Perhaps you will wonder, most sophisticated Reader, how I conceived the idea to delve into the secret lessons of the medical art that is common in China, and also to publish it among the Europeans; for it seems something strange for a religious man, and one who should spend efforts on bringing the souls of the Empire of China to God. Accept my reason for the deed, in order that some people's amazement (and perhaps rebuke) might be either forestalled or removed.

I have often wondered to myself what our Lord Jesus Christ, who had come into this world to save souls, would do. By mentioning him who is most engaged in the word and teaching, the Gospels make all things known to the People; but in order for their predictions and warnings and his holy teaching to work more deeply and persuasively into the ears and hearts of him who hears, of the Jewish People, and the Princes, what plan do you think he follows, what particular means did he use? Eternal wisdom found nothing else more effective than if he made himself a doctor of the body, that he might heal souls more easily through bodily salvation. He healed by word alone, and his word, that his utterance could benefit the lost,[19] and he convinced them of their immortality, since the immortal Physician banished death itself from mortals. In fact, he accomplished this through his miraculous healing of fevers, dropsy, paralysis, a leper, and a thousand other diseases, so that he seemed to administer salubrious medicines to their souls, and bring their nature, tainted by the poisonous consumption of the forbidden fruit and subjected to all illnesses and death itself, to an immortality of life. Not only did he want to be the Doctor, but he wanted to be called so as well, since there would be no need of a Doctor for healthy persons, but for those who were faring

---

[19] Some neat alliteration here: *ut perditis prodesse posset praedicatum*

poorly, he calls himself life, salvation, resurrection. Since that is the case, when it pleased God to separate me above my fellows and to call me through his grace to preach his word among the Nations, I endeavored constantly to shape myself to his life. Therefore, I determined that I had to follow the means for saving the Nations that was given by God. Since I found that I had succeeded among the ailing in Europe, it is clear that Physicians and those who say that they know something about this science find ready approaches—to everyone, in fact—I decided that knowledge of this skill was not useless for enriching the souls of the Chinese and penetrating their hearts. Therefore, after I applied myself to the Chinese language, and spent the same effort on Chinese characters, I endeavored to delve into their medical arts, which I did by reading a great number of Chinese Doctors. Afterwards, I endeavored to grasp the tremendous antiquity and experience and even relationships within those things[20] that they provide; then I wondered how the Wisest God not only created Peoples similar to Europeans in that farthest part of the World, but endowed them with many natural gifts and talents, riches as well as Governance, almost all arts, and especially the noblest knowledge of the art of medicine. Therefore, I thought that it should be widely publicized, for how would I hide such a great treasury? Once, Galen, while admiring the workshop of this circle, cried that no one else could have been its Craftsman but God. The royal Prophet reflected upon the structure of bones in man sometimes, and, as though he were snatched outside himself, being mindful of the thanks that were owed, he said to his Founder: "All my bones will speak, Lord, who is like you?" "It was not I," says the holy mother of the Maccabees to her sons, "that gave you a spirit and soul and life; not I that put together each of your limbs, but the Creator of the world, who fashioned the birth of man and who discovered the beginning of all things and shall restore to you your soul and life,

---

[20] *Adverti habere adeo magnam antiquitatem & experientiam, atque etiam connexionem earum rerum*, literally, "I turned to have the so-great antiquity and experience, and also the connection of these things," I think the sense is that he attempted to study all aspects of Chinese medicine as fully as possible and to understand them deeply.

Michal Boym

in his pity." Exactly as the Wisdom of God and the traces of that
life shall shine more brightly in the medicines that he left for
mortals; so too will the life of men, which he made in a certain
ineffable way to grant a rational and immortal soul to a
corruptible body; to preserve and restore it, he also bestowed the
very art of medicine. The foresight and wisdom of God shines,
so that, from this mortal life, men could recognize the author of
that immortal life. Even if men here marvel at the knowledge of
restoring life and the marvelous operations of life (which <life>
everyone loves so greatly) in Medicine; so much more would
they be forced to marvel at their Author and to praise life itself,
or him for whom all things live, and in whom we all live, move,
and exist! This was the most powerful reason for broadcasting
the newly-discovered learning of the Chinese in the Art of
Medicine,[21] in order for the Reader to be roused to the praise of
God and to marvel at his Wisdom and to long for that eternal life
which God states that he will give, when he offers medicines and
the medical arts for prolonging life, for his glory and the
expansion of good deeds. Its utility also persuaded me to
broadcast this same work for sick men to seize upon, as well as
Priests, who have the duty of purging their sins or of leading men
at the final struggle. Thus, it would be very easy for men who
are so sick, when they are put in danger, to be able to know
themselves, and for Priests to help them and give them advice
about their impending death and the care for salvation based on
the signs and judgments, which you have at this point in a much
greater quantity and with greater ease than perhaps any other
Physician would notice. A Philosopher at this point will get what
he longs to know, what the object of his search is, if he examines
those secrets which God gave to nature, and which the Chinese
received from most ancient tradition; and if he contemplates a
certain harmony and agreement between the Microcosmos and
the Megacosmos. The Mathematician will get it, too, when he
notices that the crises and his final days,[22] an accounting of

---

[21] *novum Sinarum in Arte Medica inventum*, literally, "the new thing of the
Chinese found in the Medical Art."
[22] *decretorios dies*, literally, "deciding days," in reference to the last days of
one's life.

which they tend to attribute to numbers, arise from other, more secret causes. The astrologer will get it, when he marvels that the Chinese discovered that the movement of the heavens was in accord with the course of a normal human life, which it influences with a marvelous effectiveness.

The physicist will get it when he recognizes that changes in the human body occur no differently than they do in the universe. The Physicians will get things to explore diligently, to test, observe, and reduce to practical use for men. That no one might doubt the truth of what has been said once they have read it, and partly that those Chinese who are not unaware of the Latin language of Europe might state to all the world that I have spoken truly about their Art, I have taken care for that same book to be written out in Sino-European characters, and I included a Latin translation (and in order that it be the easier to understand, I inserted some words, and not ones that I made up, but that were taken from the Chinese text of another passage, or from commentaries on that same text). Therefore, whosoever of you wish to read this book, printed without text that was finished with Chinese and Latin letters, do not put your faith in it, but reject what is false! For it is clear to me that, when the text is overlooked, many faulty ambiguities can creep in. I call you to the text, which I provide, whole and uncorrupted; but I ask that you read everything from the beginning, that you strive to memorize it, for these things are of the greatest use to understand what comes after. If you spurn the fundamentals at the outset, believe me, you will not be able to understand the final pieces, since you will not easily find an end when the thread is broken; for there is a marvelous connection between all the things which the Chinese provide, and an understanding of one depends upon the other. Therefore, everything must be read if you wish to grasp even a single lesson in this art. Note too that the manner of reading among the Chinese differs from the European way, for they begin reading from the left and then move down the edge of the page; and you will see that I have followed the second part in the book that is joined here, but I have changed the first part, and I have adapted it to the style of reading taken from Latin.

But I would like you to know, most civilized Reader, that I have taken the majority of what I have gathered in this key after much toil and hard work, based on Physicians' authentic books, those most current in the Chinese Empire, and those which, promulgated by order of the Tribunals and the Emperor himself, have been reprinted again and again. I also have many others that will need to be published, if it please God. Next, I have no doubt about the certainty of the Art, for they would not have dared to lie to the entire Empire or to force it for so many ages upon those people  at whose order those things have been published. Add too that the Art itself, or rather its foundation, is exceedingly ancient, and that new commentaries are almost in agreement with the ancient ones—and I am especially astounded at that, as if they were identical! This agreement, in the face of such a great variety of talents, the multitude of men, and any chance misfortune, can and should seem quite amazing. Then I also added the actual text of the most ancient book of all on the art of medicine, after the Chinese key, partly in order that they might take their authority from that which I mentioned, partly in order no one might have malicious feelings or be suspicious about its trustworthiness, according to how I translated it.

The style in this key is prosaic and hurried rather than stylish and elegant, for I followed, as far as I could, the manners of speaking among the Chinese; it shall be clear from reading how they differ from European styles. I was mindful of the great Augustine, who says, in the fourth book *On the Christian Doctrine*, chapter 11: it is a noteworthy characteristic of good persons to love what is true in words, not the words themselves, for what good is a golden key if it cannot open what we want? Or what hindrance is a wooden key if it can do this, when we want nothing but to lay bare what is closed.

# Another Preface, to be placed before the book of formulas

*<By the same Father>*[23]

This book that follows is a method, or rather a standard for curing ailments that is widely used among the Chinese. That most noble man and the first of the doctors discovered and assembled it, and the author, *uâm Xŏ hŏ*,[24] added it the Art of taking pulses that he passed down, and today all Chinese Doctors follow him; and in fact, even they did not learn about a sick person's pulse from the man himself, they are altogether safe, because the medicines that are here prescribed for pulses will also treat diseases, and everyone has learned through long experience that the medicines cited here produce definite healing. Therefore, if healing does not follow, they say that either it was applied inappropriately; or the pulses were not correctly identified; or this evil was in fact connected with another evil; or lastly, medicine was added to a pulse that cannot be fixed. Therefore, whoever wants to use these medicines, I beg him to train studiously and carefully in looking into and distinguishing different pulses, so that someone's rashness or inexperience does not make this book, to which I wanted to turn for the well-being of many, into a poison—not without resentment from me against the one who is undeserving.

But perhaps the names of Chinese medicines happen to be entirely unknown to you, as well as the medicines themselves, whence you conclude that it is impossible for the Europeans to use this book. Indeed, I wanted to offer a remedy for this problem, and I had in fact already proposed to compile a Chinese herbarium[25] and to describe the virtues of the medicines that they use with appropriate drawings of the plants. But since this

---

[23] Entire title of preface is a little unclear: *Alia Praefatio ante librum receptarum ponenda. Ejusdem P.*

[24] Seems like it's the name of the author, but it's unclear.

[25] A book pertaining to plants.

require a great deal of time and effort, as well as the freedom and opportunity to work, which I had not yet found, I decided to put off completing that task for another time, God willing. After I set out from China for Europe and was staying at Goa, I had written to the Friends of Macao[26] and even furnished expenses with which I could ship the medicines of the Chinese (almost all of which I had included in a catalogue) to myself in Europe. I had this in mind, that the medicines of the Chinese could be compared with those of Europe, and that ones like it and of similar efficacy could be substituted by skilled men in their place. This desire, however, could not reach its end at that time, and the wish could not achieve its outcome. But if you earnestly wish to procure the medicines that the Chinese have and which you read about here from the Merchants that leave for India or Macao, you will take care to procure them in the Chinese characters described in this book, for just as rhubarb and the Chinese radish is brought to Europe and in such great quantities, so too it is certain that other medicines could be brought—that is, those which they acquire for use in various parts of the Chinese Empire, and which are likewise gathered and sold for a pittance.

Here you may find drinks and powders and pills, for the Chinese treat all maladies by these three methods. It is necessary, however, to observe carefully those things that they say need to be observed, with an accounting of the food that they prescribe, which I have dealt with at some length at the end of the medical key.

Note too, when we talk here about weight, that China is entirely unfamiliar with the weights of Scruples, drachmas, and <tinctures>[27] that the Doctors of Europe use. Among them, a weight is used that they call the *seúm*, which is equal to the weight of a Roman shield and contains ten Julii, in almost equal parts. They call the Julian weight of each of them a *Czên*, then

---

[26] *Amicis Macaensibus*, I think *Macaensis* is a neologism meaning "of Macao."
[27] *ana* (?)

the Julius itself (that is, the *Czên*) they subdivide into ten equal parts, which they call *Fuen*: then they divide the *Fuen* into ten *lî*, and so forth.

They tend to weigh everything with these three weights, including[28] medicines and their doses.

Note too that they measure water with a large bowl and a small bowl, typically of porcelain, from which they drink either wine or *cha* or *thè*. I turned the normal goblet,[29] so it would be neither too small nor too large, and I substituted a large goblet for the bowl.

A decoction is also ordered to be made of the medicines in water, which should generally be understood so that, out of ten parts water, three are used up, and seven remain (speaking normally), unless you see something marked out in a particular passage.

Finally, the practice of treating ailments, which we have added to the end of the medical key, is as follows: When a pulse is properly recognized, and it has taken the place of a connatural[30] pulse in any of three locations (for there is no difference whether the locations are in the right- or the left-hand), check the book and take care that those medicines which are attributed to this pulse are prepared and taken. If you want to be precise, check that the pulse in that location—that is, the first or second or third location (*cún quan chě*)—is just as the sick man has found it; fashion the medicines according to the invading pulses in the first, second, or third passage, whether that be a draught, or pills, or powder, before or after food; or offer the sick person what they need to take either hot or cold, as it is prescribed there;

---

[28] *non solum alia, sed etiam...ponderure solent*, "They tend to weigh not only other things, but even..."

[29] *Ego calicem verti ordinarium*, exact meaning unclear, particularly of *verti*.

[30] *connaturalis* is a word that appears extensively throughout this book. I translate it as a cognate, "connatural," where that makes sense, but I often also translate it as "having the same nature" or "sharing the same nature." The exact sense of the Latin is sometimes unclear, because (as the author says), he is copying his understanding of Chinese stylistics.

repeat, until you see that the connatural pulse has returned.[31] I would like you to note one thing here: Since there is a great difference in the climate of Europe and China, and likewise between rice and wheat, and likewise such foods (for instance, all Chinese food and drink is hot, which is not the same in Europe) and other such things, a careful and studious doctor must take account of such a great difference in treating the ill and choosing medicines.

Therefore, think well of this little effort of mine, which has engaged me for ten full years, amid many serious tasks, and with its own starts and stops, because I felt that I would be doing something of value. Marvel at God, Reader, who has granted life to men, and wanted the mysterious creation of this very life to be thus beheld. Love God, who, when we wretched mortals are pressed by so many evils of the mind and body, which is our desert, he tends to the one and the other with remedies that are so fitting and so effective.

*Annotation on this preface to the book of formulas*

A book of Chinese formulas seems to be of little use to a European. Reason 1) Because many sorts of plants are unknown and have not yet been grown in European soil. 2) Roots and plants, even if they are dried, largely cannot be brought to Europe, because they are eaten up by worms and moths almost before they reach Macau or Batavia;[32] all the more if they are brought to Europe. 3) Based on the plants and cultivated roots themselves, a Doctor can hardly determine whether their like can be found elsewhere in Europe. It would be a chore to run all over China and look into the plants and trees when they are still alive and fresh. 4) The plants and roots which are sold in apothecaries must be prepared ahead of time with great care, some with wine, others with pure water or salt water, a salve of rice or wheat or some trifle[33]; some must be steeped with vinegar, others in a

---

[31] Very awkward

[32] *Batavia*, refers to a number of different places; usually Holland, but maybe here in reference to Jakarta, Indonesia?

[33] *parvuli*, literally, "of a little tiny <thing>."

lump of flour; some with nuts, others must be folded in with a clod of earth and allowed to rot[34] under ash and gentle fire; some with sugar-water or licorice-water, others must be drunk with the steam of boiling water and then exposed to the wind or the Sun from the ninth of the morning until the third after noon,[35] as is the case with rhubarb, which is steeped[36] nine times with water vapor and is laid out each time to be dried by the sun, so that it will keep longer and be cleansed of the pollution that it possesses, while saving its natural virtue, which, since it is so cold, actually reconstitutes itself more by fire or the sun than it loses or gives off out of doors. Likewise, for some plans and roots, the pit is removed; for others, the rind.[37] In the use of some, care must be taken against side-effects;[38] for some, certain things even need to be added to serve as vehicle for the plants, as with, for example, Ginger, and others like it. 5) Certain roots and herbs which were useful for a certain disease in ancient times have been found in modern times to be harmful or even deadly with the same malady. Finally, attention must be paid to the climate, constitution[39], food, and drink of the Chinese people, because if they apply some medicines to Southern People and others to Northerners for the same disease, what will they think needs to be done with the whole world, given that Europeans are almost broken apart?[40] Why does it seem like these formulae deserve to predominate, if pulses and the nature of the disease with respect to them are only just being understood? Medicines of every sort are not lacking Europe: medicines to ease, to comfort, to restore, to purge, to moderate,

---

[34] *mortificandae*, literally, "must be made to waste away, to grow weak," maybe fermentation?

[35] *a nona matutina usque ad tertiam pomeridianam*, "from the ninth of morning to the third of the afternoon." The concept of time measurement is explained later in the text. Time is divided into segments that do not necessarily match the idea of hours.

[36] *imbibitur*, literally, "is drunk in."

[37] *Cortex*, "hull, rind, peel, skin," etc.

[38] *a contrariis cavendum*, literally, "One must be taken from contrary / opposing things." Meaning unclear, but I think it refers to side effects.

[39] *complexionem*

[40] *fere divisis Europaeis*, "with Europeans almost divided"

to cool, to heat, etc.[41] Those disease that are already well known should be treated so that there is no need to beg them from the Chinese. But of course, this is the heart of the matter; this is the task, the effort, to properly distinguish pulses and explore their most subtle properties for this undertaking, both their use and practical applications gained from such patience,[42] as they themselves say. Therefore, if time allows, we shall attempt to make some notes about pulses (which perhaps are needed here) and to raise awareness of how Chinese Doctors talk about at least one disease (for instance, malignant fever[43]), if they talk at all, so that they can pass judgment on the rest based on a hair's-worth of evidence. Then there is the fact that things must be judged to be not unbelievable which deal with diseases, since many Doctors do not use any other treatment their whole lives than one for treating a single disease (and what was used by the Grandfathers in a family is followed by the Descendants), some focus exclusively on hectic fever, others on malignant fever, other solely on children's diseases, others only poxes,[44] others only women's diseases (which are thought to be the most challenging of all), as when diseases must be diagnosed from a pulse alone, "for, based on colors and external signs (which Physicians also want to look at) in more distinguished women, since it is not possible to see them, nothing can be gathered and determined."

---

[41] All the infinitives here are in the Latin participles: "easing medicines, comforting medicines, restoring medicines, etc."

[42] *usum experientiamque valde longanimem*, literally, "the use and very long-suffering experience / practice"

[43] *febre maligna*

[44] *solas variolas*, "only variolas," where 'variola' looks like a term for smallpox.

REVEREND FATHER MICHAŁ BOYM OF POLAND

From the Society of Jesus, from the Kingdom of Siam,

1658

# Preface to Physicians

We have brought before you, Most Famous Gentlemen, and before all Europe, from the furthest ends of the earth, the most ancient and most noble of all Physicians. If you wish to know his sort, he is Emperor, in blood and in dignity; if you wish to know his age, he is indeed much older than Avicenna, Hippocrates, Galen, and Celsus, for he is said to have lived a little more than 400 years after the flood, and began to rule in 2697 BC. Do you want to know his country? *Honám* is his Province in the Chinese Empire; *kaì fum̄* his Capital City[45], the State of *syn pi* is the Fatherland of so great a man. His name is *Hoâmti*; that is, the Yellow Emperor. This man was the first to cultivate medicines among the Chinese, and he passed his teachings in that art down to posterity, and while he was most deserving of his Empire because of his many notable deeds, he also wanted men to think well of him for this art. And so, even now, surviving in his art,[46] casting off his pride, and having learned a foreign tongue on his own, he made a journey almost to the middle of the Earth, seeking Europe, to save the life of many (something he himself lacks). But you shall say: What news does this Doctor-Emperor of yours bring? Perhaps he found more in Anatomy than Europe has known since Rondelet, Vesalius, and Bartholinus? Hardly. This man, first among Doctors, did nothing of this sort on purpose, although Chinese Doctors say that they follow him studiously in many aspects, and have even put in images those things that hide in man. I have seen their images; you would have thought them from Europe, with their detail of human Anatomy. But I could not discover anywhere whether they acquired this art from human

---

[45] The term used here is *Metropolis*.
[46] *in arte sua superstes*

dissection[47], and I would believe that the Chinese sometimes practiced dissections, since everyone recoils even from imaginary cruelty and for dead bodies. Whoever handled them, for whatever reason, would be cursed among them. Therefore, what new information does this Chinese Doctor bring? Surely he has not discovered new medicines by the practice of chemistry, or more types of plants, than Dioscorides and so many others have in Arabia, Greece, India, Europe, or Africa; men who published tremendous tomes, with plants drawn in their natural state.[48]

Not only did this Chinese Doctor excel in this area, namely by introducing many medicines and plants that were unknown to Europeans and which he gave instruction on how to use to treat ailments; but he has nothing to do with Chemistry—indeed, he will have distinction[49] between life, death, and illnesses, or something new to do with pulses. But how likely would it be that that genius of Hippocrates and those who follow him have failed to find yet everything that can be known in terms of distinctions? Who can teach more fully and more outstandingly on pulses than Galen and so many other outstanding Doctors who came after him? For it is said the most ancient Doctor, the Yellow Emperor, offers distinctions entirely different from Hippocrates; likewise, he offers knowledge of pulses entirely different from Galen, one which no one has even dreamed of. Moreover, he discovered and passed down a rationale for treating diseases that is entirely new and distinct from the European way—and all these things which I have mentioned were done almost at the time of the flood. I set these things before you, most skillful Gentlemen, along with their author, in a medical key, which I have had produced in order to crack open an Art that has lain hidden in books, described so anyone who wants can find it. This Chinese Doctor lays the foundation for distinctions between life and death in the knowledge of pulses, from which he shows "not only how to predict death or illnesses, but even circumstances or conditions

---

[47] In context, it seems like he's talking about vivisection.

[48] *ad vivum*, unclear idiom.

[49] *aphorismos*

that are caused by diseases, and you will hardly find anyone among Chinese Doctors who asks of those around him what sort of illness a sick man has, or what he suffered from, since he foretells everything after the pulse is looked into, even up to the marvelous disease,[50] and he shows what things have arisen from it or will arise.

He can even predict death, not only when it is imminent, but months, a year, or even years in advance.[51] Once, I read that Galen had made some predictions based on pulses, and in fact, had even taught how to make predictions, in case[52] that if anyone ate or toiled under some affliction and even some other disease. But in order to identify universally each and every disease based on pulses, or in order for him or another person to show how to recognize this and determine their dispositions based on that, there has been no one that I know of thus far. This Emperor alone taught this skill, in observance of whose teaching Chinese Doctors even today follow <him>, among the Chinese people and the various sorts of diseases that come from them.[53] But what, you ask, does it have to do with pulses that it has not already been discovered by Galen and others? I mentioned above what altogether different, and in fact contradictory things have not been conceived of, and although I cover these things in some detail in the Medical key, I put other things her under the net. Everyone following Galen says that you should only take the pulse in one hand; Hoâmti says both. Galen says the left hand, while Hoâmti says that one should take pulses not only in the left hand, but in the right hand first, because, of course, life begins and ends there. Galen argues that a single spot in the left hand is enough for this; Hoâmti says that three spots in the right hand are necessary to take the pulse, and the same amount in the left hand, nor does he stop there: he offers instruction on how to take and distinguish pulses in both the right and left arm, at a shallow, moderate, or deep depth (that is, on the skin and flesh;

---

[50] *miraculum morbum*, epilepsy?
[51] A somewhat free translation, but it conveys the sense.
[52] *ut si*, literally, "as if" or "in order that if"
[53] Exact meaning unclear.

in the blood and nerves; and finally in the bones), whatever pulse they may have. Moreover, he observed that, in a woman and a man, even the natural pulses in those three places differ vastly. What else? He showed that lightness and heaviness exist in pulses. Then? He taught that the measure of pulses is an infallible guide to life and illnesses, which agrees with the intervals of breaths. Galen freely admits that he does not know the length of time, although he tried over a long period to look into it. What shall I say about the natures of pulses and how they differ from each other, and about that remarkable definitive connection that has been discovered with the conditions which he foretold? What shall I say about the causes that he assigned to the differences between pulses? What about the circulation of blood and Spirits[54], and their return? What about his predictions, and his colors, sounds, tastes, scents, and fluids? What about the rest, up to the art of medicine itself? Surely the Chinese treat pulses and not diseases—no, in fact, they treat diseases through pulses; that is, when they discover that an unwholesome pulse has taken the place of a natural one,[55] they offer medicine for the unwholesome pulse, so that it either departs or returns to its natural state. How could anything be more wonderful? What shall I say about the knowledge of pulses; namely, how pulses produce, increase, attack, and destroy themselves in turn? But whoever wants to know this and other things, let him take the medical key and consider every part of it. I offer one bit of advice, that those who approach this Chinese chamber not let the strange appearance of things trouble their mind. After you see everything, then you may pass judgment on the whole work and its elements.

But whoever does not follow the reasoning and causes for everything that we relate, let him look to experience itself and

---

[54] *Spiritus*, precise meaning in this book unclear. It is always contrasted with blood, but seems to be something since disproven (like humors). It can often mean "breath," but the book seems to prefer a different word (*spiratio*) for the process of breathing.

[55] *pro naturali irrepsisse contranaturalem...pulsum*, "that a pulse against nature has snuck in in place of a natural <pulse>"

remember, that that which has been in use for so many centuries, which was proven in the most flourishing and greatest Empire, which even now is extremely vibrant, such as the Bavarians, English, Portuguese, and other nations that have visited Chinese ports can bear witness, cannot fail to have its own causes, and secure ones at that, which the Art of foretelling diseases relies upon.

Come now, Most Renowned Men, and practice this Art yourselves according to your own genius! And just as your ancestors gave much clarity and glory to these studies and pursuits of theirs, which they received from Galen and Hippocrates, likewise, strive to share your ancestor's praise, refine this work, illustrate it, and complete it, so that we may hear in time that these Chinese pulses, already made clearer by Europeans, resonates over the whole World. We conclude, and we ask you to defend this effort of ours, however it may turn out, against the uncouth and the critics; and finally, for you to pray to GOD Almighty, that he not allow this people, whom he wanted to be thus trained in the art of treating bodies, to be any longer lacking in skilled Doctors of the soul and in heavenly medicines, with the help of Him by whose suffering we have been restored, who is the salvation, life, resurrection of all things, to whom alone belongs the honor and Empire for ages upon ages.

-Reverend Father Michał

REVEREND FATHER

MICHAŁ BOYM OF POLAND

From the Society of Jesus,

# The Medical Key to
# the Doctrine of the Chinese on Pulses

# CHAPTER ONE

*What the cause of life and health is in man*

The ancient Chinese believed that a living and healthy man is made up of a certain conjunction, almost agreement, between two qualities, which they call *yâm* and *iñ*.[56] By *yâm*, they mean the primordial heat; by *iñ*, they mean radical wetness.[57] They say that the Spirit and the blood, both mentioned in the human body, are the vehicles of radical wetness and primordial heat (for which reason *yâm* and *iñ* are in fact designated by the same words among the Chinese), and if they agree with each other appropriately and proportionally, they say that they also have primordial heat and radical wetness of the finest order, and thus perfect life and health for man exists and is maintained.

The Chinese state that *Jin* (by which term they mean man, which they also express with this character ) is made from *yam*, whose mark is , and in whose mark is joined together.

From those two written characters comes that Chinese Character, or rather, the entire meaning of "man," and in this way, from the symbol for the word *yâm* combined with the symbol for *iñ*, comes the word meaning "man" in Chinese, *yâin*. Thus, the argument is made that the definite life and health of man comes from those qualities which are jointly shared with each other in the human constitution: *yam*, primordial heat, and *in*, radical wetness; but in the meantime, it first changes based on the unharmonious conjunctions of the aforementioned qualities and their violent separation, and grows weak; then it dissolves, and at last is extinguished. Using almost the same

---

[56] Technically, *in* has a line above the 'n.' From here on, I will not provide every tone-marker or accent in the Chinese transliterations.
[57] The Latin terms for "primordial heat" and "radical wetness" are *color primigenius* and *(h)umidum radicale*. Other sources have translated *humidum radicale* as "radical moisture."

reasoning, the Chinese character ⟨figure⟩, when it is separated into its two parts, ⟨figure⟩ and ⟨figure⟩, fully loses all sense of "man."

They think that those two primordial qualities are hidden in the chief organs[58] and intestines of the human body, as though they are at their source, and thus spread to the rest of the body; and based on those things, according to the nature of that from which they emanate, each part of the body receives life and health, action and operation, each according to their own need.[59]

If, at some time, they find that the unchanging qualities that we just discussed in the organs and intestines are changed,[60] either entirely or in part, then diseases arise, strength and life fail, and death looms large. But on the other hand, if they find them whole and in agreement with one another appropriately in their proper turn, they gather certainly that the man is healthy, is at full strength, and will have a long life.

Then it is clear among Chinese Doctors that the cause of life and health in man comes from *in*, radical wetness; and *yam*, primordial heat, just as life (does which emanates from them through Spirits and blood) when it acts upon the person's entire body and each of its components in due measure, just as it guides, penetrates, shapes, and invigorates them.

---

[58] *membra*, literally, "limbs," but based on context it is likely best translated as "organs." I am unsure what the technical difference is between organs (*membrum*) and intestines (*intestini*).

[59] *pro sua quamque exigentia*, "according to their own smallness

[60] *immutatus* can be "unchanging" or "changed", so this could also read "...that the qualities that we just discussed in the organs and vitals are changed, are altered..."

## CHAPTER TWO

*What the seat of life is in man*

The Chinese divide the parts of the human body into *Câm* and *fu*. The first word applies to the organs, the latter to the intestines.

The chief organs, in which the *iñ*, the radical wetness, particularly reside, are six in number.

On the left side: *Sin,* the heart; *kan*, the liver; *Xin*, the kidneys. On the right side: *fì*, the lungs; *pi*, the spleen; *mím múcú*, the gate of life.

Likewise, the intestines (or the 'inner parts,' if you prefer), in which the *yâm*, the primordial heat, particularly reside, are six in number.

On the left side: *Siáo châm*, which are properly called the small intestines; *fu*, the gall bladder;[61] *pam kuam*, the ureters.[62]

On the right side: *tá châm*, that is, what are properly called the large intestines; *quey*, the stomach; *Sin crao*, the third part of the body.

The Chinese also divide the human body into three parts. The first is the uppermost part, called the *Xam crao*, and it is that which extends from the head to the chest. The middle is *chum crao*, from the chest to the waist, or the navel. The third and lowest, the *hia crao* and *san crao*, extends from the navel to the bottom of the feet.

The organs in Chinese are called *Câm*, which means "to store away," for they store away cither food, or blood, or fluids, or humors, or spirits. They call the intestines *fu*, which is the same

---

[61] *folliculum fellis*, literally, "the sack of gall," although *fel, fellis* is alone to describe the gall bladder as well.

[62] *ureteres*, something to do with the urinary tract, although I do not know if it corresponds directly to the modern medical understanding of "ureters."

as 'hall' or 'colony,'[63] because those things which are stored away in the organs apply are carried to the inner parts of the organs, just like they are brought to halls or colonies. But since they found that the chief parts, (sometimes the organs, sometimes the intestines) engage with each other to a great degree because of their proximity and serve one another in turn, so have they connected individual elements, like the intestines, to individual organs.

And so, on the left side, they connected the small intestines to the heart,[64] the gall bladder to the liver, the ureters to the kidneys. On the right side, the large intestines to the lungs, the stomach to the spleen, the third part of the body to the gate of life. They state that the qualities of radical wetness and primordial heat, qualities that are inherent in them from the outset, reside and are kept in these organs and entrails, and that they spread life throughout the entire body according to their varying dispositions through various motions, spirits, and actions; for the first Doctors among the Chinese did this with the utmost care, so that they had examined the natural temperaments and dispositions of the organs and entrails individually. After they had learned that they could understand with certainty all of these things (particularly their agreement and disagreement) based on daily measuring of pulses (exactly like skilled lyrists, after they have explored the strings of their lyre, learn the harmonious or dissonant character of those strings and the whole lyre), they themselves handed down to posterity a most beautiful knowledge of pulses. This knowledge has been maintained and has thrived, even up until modern times, and we shall reveal it below, God willing.

The *con*, satisfied to have found the sources and origins of life in the six organs and six conjoined intestines, sought certain indications of these things throughout the whole human body.

---

[63] *atrium sive colonia*

[64] Literally, *cordis membro*, "the organ of the heart." All of these pairings use this clunky expression, which I have translated more smoothly for readability.

And after they had found various things in different parts of the body, they learned that there appear certain signs of life and health, of diseases, and of death, particularly in the head of both the organs and intestines. They call these sing *heu cyé*, which we shall hereafter call the "external indicators of the current condition."[65] Furthermore, they say that the external sensory organs (which are seen everywhere, particularly on the head) are bound to the sources of life—the organs and intestines. The tongue to the heart, the nose to the lungs, mouth to spleen, ears to kidneys, eyes to liver. Indeed, because of the variety of colors which show themselves in the forehead, eyes, nose, and ears; based on the distinction and variety of the tastes which the tongue either perceives or seeks out; even that of the voice which the patient produces, they boast—not in vain—that they can determine the times of life and death with reasonable certainty. Thus, based on the six organs and the same number of intestines that have been discussed (which are twelve sources; or rather, if we number them according to the intestines that are joined to the organs, there are six sources total), they argue that life is distributed throughout the rest of the body, and even into the external sense organs, through radical wetness and primordial heat. In whatever way the organs and intestines are variously moderated and still submit to many different dispositions, in the same way the organs that are connected to each other impact other parts of the body which are subordinated to them and near them in many different ways.

In the meantime, note that the Chinese only say sometimes that there are six organs, sometimes five—that is, the liver, heart, lungs, spleen, and kidneys; because, of course, the kidneys are double, insofar as there is one on the left side of the body which has the name 'kidney,' and one on the right side which is called the 'gate of life.' Again, the Chinese say at times that there are six intestines (which, as we mentioned above, they connect to the same number of organs), at other times five—the small and large intestines, the gall bladder, the ureters, the stomach; the *quīa Sañ Ciao*, the third part of the body, is more on the outside,

---

[65] *externos temporariae constitutionis indices*

but some parts are inside. As for what is called the third part, it happens to be the sixth intestine, although it does not have the appearance of what is properly called an intestine, because it is the place of the internal spirits, so it is also connected to the gate of life which produces them.

Based on what has been said, it follows that the seat of life in man in twelve sources, six, I say, the fonts of life.

It remains for us to explain how the chief organs distribute radical wetness throughout the whole body and its individual parts; and likewise how the chief intestines do so with primordial heat, each one according to its own nature; or, what is the same thing, through what paths or routes of life (which resides variously in the individual organs and intestines) it is conveyed for the many and various operations of the body in the blood and spirits, as though it were conveyed by vehicles.

## CHAPTER THREE

*Through what paths or routes the principal organs and the principal intestines (that is, those which are the seats or fonts of life and health, together with the rest of the human body, share life and health.*[66]

Chinese physicians assign three organs to the right side, and three intestines that are connected to them; the same number appear on the left, as we have already shown in the previous chapter. From the organs of radical wetness (*iñ*), and from the intestines of primordial heat (*yâm*), they describe how the virtues, intermingling with each other, spread throughout the rest of the body in a unified effort. These are the paths:

From the left, they say that the noblest organ, the heart, pours[67] radical wetness to the hands, and this route is called (*xoá xán yn kím*), "the path of the lesser radical wetness to the hands from the heart."[68] Connected to the heart, the small intestines pour primordial heat by the same path, and so they call this conduit of heat, (*xeú tái jám kím*), "the path of the great radical heat of the hands from smaller intestines."

Two sources are supplied from those two paths, and they make up a single font of life (and so it is with everything else).

The liver distributes radical wetness to the feet, and they call this channel (*Co kiue yn kim*), "the defective[69] path of the radical

---

[66] There is no closing parenthesis here.

[67] *derivatur*, actually passive (literally, "the heart is flowed"), but I think the author is using the equivalent of middle voice ("the heart pours from itself...")

[68] *manuum a corde diminuti humidi radicalis via*, "the path of the hands from the heart of the diminished radical wetness," I think *manuum* is a subjective genitive with *via* ('the hand's . This holds true throughout this chapter.

[69] *defectuosi*, from *defectus*, "lack," "failing," and the suffix –*osus*, meaning "full of." This derives ultimately from the verb *deficio*, which is used later of different classes of pulses, and I think they are related.

wetness of the feet from the liver." And because primordial heat flows to the feet from the gall bladder like with the liver, it is called (*Cô xiáo jám kím*), "the path of diminished heat from the gall bladder to the feet." To the feet again, radical wetness travels from the kidneys; and so they call it (*Co Xáo ym kím*), the path of diminished[70] radical wetness from the kidneys to the feet. Likewise, (*co taí jam kim*), the path of the great primordial heat from the ureters to the feet, because primordial heat advances to the feet from the ureters, which are themselves connected to the kidneys. And so the routes on the left side of the body have been described.

Now, on the right side of the body, the lungs, they say, pour radical wetness down to the hands, that is, by (*Xeu taì yn kím*), the path of great radical wetness from the lungs to the hands. Likewise, primordial heat, which travels from the large intestines (which are connected with the lungs), works its way into the hands by the route called (*Xem iâm mîm kîm*), the path of pure and bright primordial heat from the large intestines to the hands.

They show that radical wetness flows from the spleen to the feet, and that primordial heat flows to the feet from the stomach, which is next to the spleen. This route is (*co iâm mím kim*), the path of pure and bright primordial heat from the stomach to the feet; the other is (*co tái yñ kim̄*), the path of the great radical wetness from the spleen to the feet.

Finally, radical wetness proceeds from the gate of life to the hands, and it is called (*xeu kiūe yn kim̄*), the path of failing radical wetness from the gate of life to the hands. The third part of the body which is connected to it gives primordial heat to the feet by the path to which they gave the name (*Xeu Xao iam̄ kim̄*),

---

[70] *diminuti*, literally meaning "broken up," "shattered," from the verb *diminuo*. I have tried to translate it throughout as "diminished." Many terms used in this text seem to be technical medical terminology; in those cases, I will indicate the word and what translation I prefer for it.

that is, "the path of diminished heat from the third part of the body to the feet."

Following this scheme, the whole human body, fully endowed with radical wetness and primordial heat, in the opinion of the Chinese, draws strength and life from these very things, which[71] certainly emanates from its own origins and fonts through those routes which we have already discussed.

There are twelve paths to twelve origins: six organs, the foundations of radical wetness; and six intestines, the vents of primordial heat, like twelve hills. They draw down an equal number of vital fonts. Only six of these fonts are commonly counted, because, of course, each one of the aforementioned organs and intestines pours life, which results from the aforementioned qualities, through the mentioned paths throughout the human body, only by some sort of joint agreement and by the identical inlet.

Therefore, whoever recognizes the nature and disposition of these six fonts, or perhaps twelve sources, will no doubt have beheld the entire condition of the organs and intestines. Besides that, whoever will have tracked the dispositions of the twelve paths and their inherent natures, their increases and decreases, as well as their changes and other qualities, they will easily be able to surmise and predict faults in organs and intestines, their diseases, and their failure.

Now, though, we must state how the Chinese understand the nature and characters of the six fonts of life, or the twelve sources (the organs and intestines, I mean); and the qualities of their twelve flowing paths, both natural and preternatural.[72]

---

[71] *quae*, I think it refers to "life," *vitam*, but it might also refer to "scheme," *ratione*.

[72] *praeter naturales*, written as one word later in the book. Literally meaning "beyond what is natural" or "separate from what is natural."

## CHAPTER FOUR

*What is the nature, what the dispositions and qualities of the twelve paths which are led from the twelve origins, and which convey life and health throughout the human body?*

The Chinese reason that the Elements of the world came from the heavens and the qualities connected with the heavens, that is *yâm*, heat, and *yñ*, wetness (two of which are produced from *t'ai kiě*, which means chaos or an unformed substance); they argue that there are no fewer than five: Earth, Metals, Water, Trees (Air), and Fire. The reasoning for this is that all things that are seen and which exist in the universe are held in this group of five,[73] so they are called 'Elements,' as though they are the first sorts of things to which all other things are reduced.

The human body, its organ and intestines, do not consist of simple things, but mixed. Yet because they had found in the mixture and dispositions of these things, in each of the organs and intestines, that any one quality of a single Element predominates above the rest, they gave the names of individual Elements to individual organs and intestines. So for the left side of the human body, the most exceptional organ, the heart, because it is possessed of a red or fiery color, and likewise a bitter taste, because it seethes and boils beyond all the other organs, and likewise with the small intestines (*hò*) connected to the heart, they gave them the name the Element of fire.

They assert that both things belong to the Southern region, the area called *ligua*, because in their opinion the Element of fire resides there as though its in its proper place, and boils very powerfully in the summer (and thus it happens that the heart produces its own qualities especially in the summer).

They assign to the liver the name and nature *mo*, that is, that of trees, plants, air, and winds; they do likewise to the liver because of its blue color and its somewhat sour nature. They teach that

---

[73] *quinario*

both things pertain to the east, and *Xin,* the region of the heavens, because the power of growth and the winds are produced there, just like in their native place, and because they release their powers more fully in the spring (where the dispositions of the liver then are particularly noticeable).[74]

They wish for the *Xui,* that is, the element of water, to be included among the kidneys and the ureters, because a certain briny taste in them, and their somewhat blackish color, and particularly coldness (radical wetness), all take the chief place, and so they put those things are under the *qua kien* part of the heavens to the North, because the Element of water freezes there because of great cold, and so in the winter the kidneys produce fuller indications and effects. On the right side, they said that the lungs, on account of their dryness and because they have a somewhat parched taste and because they have a whitish color (just as the large intestines do), are ruled by the *kin,* that is, the element of metal.

Both are subject to the west and the *qua kiuen* portion of the sky. And because they think that metals are made during the Autumn, so they say that the lungs and the large intestines assert their power and give signs of it chiefly at that time of year.

They have given the name *tu,* that is, 'earth,' to the spleen, because of its quality of warmth, its sweet taste, and yellow color. For the same reason, they say that the stomach, which is connected to the spleen, is earthen.

They have stated that both are located in the middle of the four elements under the region of heaven (they call it *gua ken*), and that they assert their powers in the third month (from the standpoint of the four seasons in any given year).

They place the gate of life, and the third part of the body connected to it, under the Master of fire as well as water, and so

---

[74] *unde hepatis affectiones tunc maxime spectantur,* awkward phrasing.

they think that its takes qualities from the heart and kidneys and distributes what it has taken.

Have distributed the names of the Elements according to this scheme, and having observed the mastery of Elemental qualities in the individual organs and intestines of the human body, they observed how in this greater world to produce or encourage in turn things that fight less amongst themselves (the Elemental symbols); and likewise, how to destroy or corrupt dyssymbols[75] and then bring about shared changes or impressions between them. In a similar manner, they determined that either the exact same virtues of the elements, or at least not dissimilar ones, as well as the particular accomplishment of each one, were present in the organs and intestines and the paths that lead away from them. For, just as in the sublunary[76] sphere (they say), we see in a certain, definitive way, that plants or trees are produced from water, and fire from plants, but fire leaves the earth ashen, and earth is the creator of metals. Then again, metals produce or express water, and water a tree, and so on in a cycle.[77] Thus, they teach everywhere that the same cycle is accomplished in the body of man (whom the wise have rightly called the "microcosm[78]").

Since the kidneys, a watery organ, share watery qualities with the liver, an arboreal organ, which <qualities> it afterwards accomplishes or somehow converts to its own nature, then the arboreal kidney in the same way shares its qualities with the fiery heart; likewise, the fiery heart and the gates of life share their fiery natures with the earthly natures of the spleen and stomach; the spleen and stomach share their earthy qualities with the lungs, which are metallic in nature; the lungs share their metallic

---

[75] *dyssymbola*, an invented word, from the Greek δυσ- , "difficult", and σύμβολον, "token," "sign." Maybe "anti-symbol" or "misrepresentation"?

[76] *sublunari*, literally, "being under the moon." It is cognate with the archaic English "sublunary," which means "belonging to this world" (in contrast with a higher spiritual world).

[77] *in orbem*

[78] μικροκόσμον

qualities with the watery kidneys, and from these the qualities of things submit again to the arboreal liver, and so forth.

But on the other hand, just as the Element of water diminishes or even extinguishes the Element of fire,[79] so too do the cold qualities of the kidneys either lessen, change, or entirely suffocate the heat of the heart. The disposition of the liver, which we called 'subtle,' is damaged by the metallic virtue of the lungs; and just as earth tinges and suffocates water, in the same way does the spleen, abounding in earthly qualities, overwhelm or even destroy the watery disposition of the kidneys.

Therefore, if we look over how the Elements or Elementary qualities that are contained in organs and intestines affect, change, restore, increase, diminish, destroy, or corrupt themselves in turn, we shall easily come to understand their natural statuses and dispositions; and indeed, the preternatural <statuses and dispositions> of the twelve paths, and the same number of their sources (meaning the organs and intestines); and thus we shall recognize a thousand sorts of diseases, and even death itself, long before they occur.

But since we showed that it was possible to understand it through the twelve paths, the six organs, and the six intestines; and that the twelve paths reveal the source (both their own and of the others), or the dispositions of the six fonts of life, through their inherent Elementary qualities,[80] it was worth the effort to explain how to investigate the natural or unnatural state of the Elementary qualities in the organs and intestines, and <the state> of their paths.

---

[79] *aquae Elementum igneum*, I think this is zeugma, with *Elementum* being both the subject of the verbs (*aquae Elementum*) and the object (*Elementum igneum*).

[80] The author is having a lot of play here with the reflexive pronoun; the exact reference of some of the words for "their" is unclear.

## CHAPTER FIVE

*How the Elementary qualities of twelve paths in the human body, and their characters and dispositions, natural or preternatural, can be definitively determined.*

It has been taught, not only among the Chinese but also among Europeans, that human life consists of radical wetness and primordial heat. The Chinese want them stored first in the six organs, then in the six intestines, and from there to be distributed to the rest of the body along twelve paths. The characters and dispositions of the organs and intestines, they argue, cannot be traced out except along those same twelve paths, along which radical wetness and primordial heat are carried throughout the entire body. But they have determined with certainty that the paths and their heads (or rather, their beginnings) can be recognized through Elementary qualities, but that these qualities can only be recognized from pulses; this is their logic.

The pulse originates in the veins from motion; but the motion which exists in the veins comes from the flow and descent of spirits and blood. Finally, the ebb and flow of spirits and blood (of which blood is the vehicle for radical wetness, spirit the vehicle for primordial heat) direct the entire body through the twelve paths from the twelve origins (that is, the six organs and six intestines), and put each of its parts in motion.

But if it is necessary even to instigate all that creates movement, and but that which moves should either recede or stand still, it certainly follows that the pulse results from a movement that is produced by such movers and movements. Therefore, since Spirit and blood move parts of the body and drive them on as they flow down and are themselves thus moved, no pulse can fail to be from them.[81]

---

[81] *non potest ab his non aliquis pulsus existere,* "not any pulse cannot exist from these things."

Knowledge of pulses, then, is mandatory; and if we have examined their nature and differences well, we will understand the Elementary qualities that are inherent in the twelve paths; as well as their affections that are driven in the motion of blood and spirits; and thus, I say, the very organs (from which the twelve sources set out) and intestines, and the condition and dispositions of all of them. Then, when the variable surplus or deficiency[82] of Elementary qualities is understood (which are, of course, the cause of the variety in pulses), we shall know the different conditions of the paths and of the entire body. Moreover, based on connatural pulses, we will be able to surmise also the natural condition of the Elementary qualities, of blood (which transports radical wetness), of spirits (which carry primordial heat), and of the twelve path and sources; and the life and well-being of the entire human body. In order to speak with the Chinese, we can pursue the various surpluses or deficiencies in blood and spirits based on the different pulses, and thus predict countless different sorts of organs, and even impending death.

Nevertheless (they say), only he who knows how to maintain and strengthen the connatural pulses in the human body—or to bring them back and restore them, preternatural and unchanged, to their original condition, by the application of medications—only he will be able to maintain life, look into one's health, and cure diseases. For they understand one's condition[83] based on pulses that have been restored to their proper, natural condition, likewise <they understand> that the twelve paths returned to

---

[82] *vel excessu vel defectu*, both of these words appear in various form throughout the text, especially as participles: *excedentes*, "exceeding," and *deficientes*, "failing." I have translated *excessus* and *excedentes* variously (usually as "surpassing," "surplus," or "excess"), and likewise with *defectus* and *deficientes* (usually as "deficient," "deficiency," or "lack"). In general, they refer to too much (*excessus*) or too little (*defectus*) of whatever is in question.

[83] *statum*, translated variously as "status," "condition," "disposition," etc. It seems to be used synonymously with other similar Latin words (*constitutio, dispositio*, etc.) which are translated similarly.

their primeval state[84]; and likewise, life is borne by those inborn qualities in spirits and blood, when they are properly moderated; and the twelve sources that have been mentioned often distribute it[85] throughout the body.

Therefore, knowledge of pulses is absolutely essential. But since they are motions, or at least are accomplished by movement in the veins, and motion and move-ability suppose both place and time,[86] but here, there has only been explanation of how the Elementary qualities are transported from the six organs and six intestines throughout the whole body and how they move its individual parts; so we must look into the place and time at which motion takes place, and then the pulse from the motion; that is, at what parts of the body the pulse must be taken, and by what standard of time it must be measured, so that a clear and defined understanding of pulses may then be gained; and from this knowledge, <a clear and defined understanding may be gained> of the disposition of blood and spirits, of the elementary qualities, of the twelve paths, and of the same number of sources (that is, the six fonts of life), of the organs and intestines, of course, and finally of radical wetness and primordial heat, and (what are produced by these two things) of diseases and wellness, death and life.

---

[84] Grammar and meaning unclear.

[85] i.e., life.

[86] *motus autem & mobile tam locum quam tempus supponat*, exact meaning of *supponat* unclear ("put under," "put in the place <of>")

## CHAPTER SIX

*What are the more suitable pulse-locations[87] in the human body to explore the Elementary qualities of the twelve paths.*

I have discovered the pulse-locations in the human body, described just like in the Chinese Medical books; I faithfully add them below, with both the verbatim text itself and a commentary on it.

1. *Feu pe*, that is, swimming[88] whiteness (so the pulse-locations are called) are behind the ears; they approach the place where hair ends, to a measure of one finger.[89]

Commentary: A song speaks about the remiss pulse[90], you will find the aforementioned pulse-locations behind the brain at the very joint of the neck, down to the third vertebrae in the backbone.

2. Text: *san ciao*, that is, the three parts of the human body, are thus called pulse-locations.

The range of the uppermost part of the body is from the top of the head to the uppermost mouth of the stomach; the range of the middle part is from the uppermost mouth of the stomach to the lower mouth of the belly; the range of the third, or lowest

---

[87] *loca pulsuum*, "places of pulses." There are many similar genitive constructions, none of which have a fully satisfying single translation. I have translated many as hyphenated phrases (e.g., *pulmonum via*, "lung-path") in an attempt to avoid excessive clumsiness, but I also sometimes translate them with other prepositions ("the path for the lungs").

[88] *natans*, literally, "swimming" or "floating." There is an old English adjective, "natant," that could work here, but I have opted instead to translate variously as "swimming" or "floating," as seems most appropriate.

[89] *ad unam digiti mensuram*, "to one measure of a finger."

[90] *pulsu remisso*, "sent-back pulse." The exact meaning of *remissus* is unclear; the word has multiple translations (the most general of which seems to be "slackened"), but it seems like a technical term here. I will try to translate it with the cognate "remiss," unless it seems totally inappropriate in context.

part, runs from the lower mouth of the stomach, just under a middle-finger's length, straight to the soles of the feet.

3. Text: *ki múen*, that is, the gate of the extremities,[91] is the name of two pulse-locations. In women, the outermost part of their hanging nipples corresponds to the inner bone; in men and those who have smaller breasts, the pulse can be taken with a single finger. If the person is fat, it is taken with a two-finger measure below the breasts, but if they are rather thin, a measure of one and a half fingers.

4. Text: *ki hai*, that is, the sea of spirits, is thus called a pulse-location. Moreover, the measurement is taken with one and a half fingers below the middle finger.[92]

Commentary: It is called sea of spirits because in men, the repository, or sea, of seminal spirits is there.

5. Text: *tan tien*, that is, the reddened field, is thus a location. It is three finger-measures away from the navel, near *quan yuen* location—that is, the source of limits.

6. Text: *quan yuen*, that is, the source of limits. Thus is the pulse-location called which is below the name by three knuckles and a little bit more.

Commentary: This is the vein-location, which, running from the small intestines and the path of diminished radical wetness and primordial heat in the feet, is the gate, the root and foundation of the human body;[93] ultimately, the accumulation of seminal spirits.

---

[91] *extremorum porta*, "gate of outermost things."
[92] "Fingers," "scruples," and the like seem to be older measuring systems, the moder equivalents of which I do not know. It seems like the author is dividing each "finger" into ten separate parts and using those subdivisions as a standard of measurement.
[93] Grammar unclear

7. Text: *Gin im*, that is, the crossroads of man.[94] It is a so-called pulse-location and is in the left hand,[95] ahead of the boundary (which is the middle pulse), at a single part of a finger-measure (which they divide into ten parts).

Commentary: It is the seat of the liver and gall bladder. If nearly the same <pulses> are found in this pulse-location as in the place of the kidneys, it is a sign that the kidney and gall bladder are stricken with cold. Likewise, this place and the following location are called *ki keu*; that is, the mouth of Spirits. Both are subject to the lung-path of great radical wetness.

The emperor says: *Giu im* (the location's name) indicates the pulse of the stomach in the same way. Its seat is in the left hand, ahead of the boundary, at a single part of a finger-measure. Likewise, in both parts of the throat, on the right and the left, the cavity *gin im*[96] is found. The seat *gin im* is subject to the path of great radical wetness for the lungs. The hollowness *ciu im*[97] is underneath the path of pure and bright primordial heat for the stomach, or rather for the feet. Thus, *giu im* is said to also denote the pulse of the stomach.

8. Text: *ki keu*: that is, the mouth of Spirits. The location thus named is in the right hand, ahead of the boundary, or rather, the middle pulse, by a single finger-measure.

Commentary: It is the seat of the spleen and the stomach; if pulses are intense and full, it is seen that those organs are cut out of food. Why, the emperor says, does only the mouth of Spirits have mastery over five organs in the human body? Kipeus responds: the stomach is a sea of liquid and solid nourishment, and the great source of six intestines. The five tastes[98] of

---

[94] *hominis obviatio*; *obviatio* has multiple meanings, including "affability" or "openness."

[95] *in sinistra manu*, maybe means here "left-hand side"?

[96] Exact grammar with undeclinable Chinese nouns uncertain.

[97] Maybe *giu im*?

[98] *sapores*, literally, "taste" or "flavor," but I think here means something like "essence." Exact meaning unclear.

nourishment, which are taken by mouth, are merely hidden in the stomach as they nourish the five Spirits.[99] The mouth of Spirits shows the path of great radical wetness, just as it also does the spleen. The spirits and tastes of the five organs and six intestines arise from the stomach, are changed, and after being changed, appear in this pulse location called *ki keu*.

*Giu, im*, and *ki keu* are detected on both sides of the hill,[100] and they seem to imitate a collaboration, or rather a union, that is shared between heaven and earth: they are, at last, the gates of the pulses, either as they begin or end.

9. Text, *tai chum*: that is, great penetration. Two so-called pulse locations are in the two feet, behind the concavity of the big toe,[101] at a distance of two fingers'-breadths, in the very middle of the sole of the foot. Those are the very pulses that occur there.

Commentary: Some men want to mark that space as being only the span of one-and-a-half finger-measures.

From this pulse, the path is identified which leads defective radical wetness from the liver to the feet; and when you take the pulse in these places, you can certainly assume that a man is definitely alive if the pulse still endures. But if it stops, he is very nearly departed. Therefore, those locations are called the doorways of life and death.

10. Text: *tai ki*, that is, the great gulf.[102] Two pulse-locations each are called this; they are found at the side of the feet, above the heel-bone.[103]

Commentary: They reveal the path of diminished radical wetness, from the kidneys to the feet. Men have the

---

[99] Grammar / meaning unclear.

[100] *in collo utrinque*, "on the hill on both sides"

[101] *pollicis averticulum*, not sure what *averticulum* means. Something like "small concavity"?

[102] *lacuna*, meaning "hole," "gap," "ditch." Often used in literature of a piece missing from a text.

[103] *os calcanei*, could also be "mouth of the heel."

aforementioned pulse locations in their left foot, women in the right foot. Because the pulse of the kidneys is the same as that of the gate of life, so too are the markers of life and death indicated here. A sick man, then, if he has a pulse in that place because of his illness, is understood to still be alive; but if he is entirely lacking that pulse, it means that he is dead. Thus, these pulses are called the gates of life.

11. *Chum yam*, that is, the paths of primordial heat, intersect each other in turn. They are also called *hocy juuen*, that is, the fonts of accumulations,[104] and they exist at the surface of the foot, at a distance of five finger-measures between the bones, where the pulse is taken by going back from above, not in the bend itself (or rather, the hollow gulf), but at a distance of three finger-measures from it.

Commentary: It is the path of pure primordial heat—rather, the path of the stomach. Man takes spirits from Sustenance; sustenance is sent down to the stomach; the stomach disperses the tastes (spirits) among the five organs and intestines. The spirits, moreover, which are fairly pure, resolve into blood, for the spirits (wet) must be separated when they are fairly thick. Then, the purer thing, which is called *ym*, works its way into the veins and becomes blood. Which is carried outside the veins is called *quêy*; and there are hot spirits, which travel back and forth outside and inside veins. Through blood and spirits, the radical wetness and primordial heat are conveyed to all parts of the body and all its innermost nooks in something like a circular orbit, and they run through one another and are thoroughly mixed.

Moreover, because the stomach is a sea of solid and liquid sustenance, and thus furnishes the substance for all spirits, it is mastered by its various qualities and newly-arisen affections, at four times during the year, and thus the pulses of spirits should be perceptible[105] at the same times.

---

[104] *coacervationum*

[105] *percipi*, literally, "to be perceived," "to be recognized." I translate *percipio* frequently here as "perceptible," as it sounds better in a didactic

And those spirits are the foundation of the stomach and the seed of all other things, because they change not only diseases (which tend to move during the four seasons of the year[106]), but they are also the particular causes of life and death; thus, it is appropriate to take two pulses for any sick person in the *Chum yam* locations, and to examine carefully whether they do or do not contain stomach-spirits, and thus to make a judgment about life and death.

12. Text: *Fum fu*, that is, the city of winds; and it is called by another name, *Xe' puèn*, the root of the tongue. It is at the bottom of the back of the skull, where the hairline ends, from which a pulse can be taken from above, by taking it at a space of a single finger-measure.

Commentary: The flesh of the large nerves, declining towards those parts during times of malignant fever, tend to produce related[107] pulses and to emerge from the part of the head that we've already mentioned.

*See the figure for this Chinese example of what was said already, in the first Table of the Appendix, note 1.*

It will now be useful to explore whether or not, out of these cavities that we have mentioned, there are some which can indicate the 12 paths of the 12 sources and the elementary qualities that are inherent in them.

Indeed, the first of the above-mentioned locations (and the pulse behind the ears that is found in it) only indicates the path of diminished primordial heat for the hands—that is, the path of third part of the body.

---

context ("the pulse is found under these circumstances..." vs. "the pulse is perceptible under these circumstances...")

[106] *quattor anni temporibus*, literally, "in the four times of the year."

[107] *relatos*, an adjective with many meanings, the precise one here is unclear. I have, as throughout, opted for the cognate.

They count those locations as three parts of the body,[108] but they do not state that the pulses belong to the same <three parts>.[109]

The third location in the hands proves itself the path of pure heat in the large intestines.

The fourth and fifth location does not seem to mark out any path.

The sixth location, *quān yuên*, "the origin of the limit," marks its source through the path of diminished radical wetness in the feet on to the kidneys.

The seventh location in the left hand indicates the liver and gall bladder.

The eighth location, in the right hand, indicates the path of the spleen and stomach.

The ninth location in the feet indicates the path of defective radical wetness—that of the liver.

The tenth location in the feet marks out the path of diminished radical wetness—that of the kidneys.

The eleventh provides the path of pure primordial heat; that is, the path of the stomach.

The final location, *fūm fú*, leads to a partial understanding of the state of the lungs.

But since it is clear from this introduction that not all paths and the origins of paths are opened from the pulse-locations we went through, if nothing further is brought forth, it will again be necessary to look into other pulse-locations, so that once these things are understood, the elementary qualities of the twelve

---

[108] *illi*, could describe any number of things—the path, the location (*locus*), the primordial heat. Exact meaning unclear.

[109] Strange grammar. The author seems to use genitives as a workaround for the verb "to have": here, *non declarant earundem pulsus*, "they do not declare the pulses of the same <three parts>" = "they do not say that the pulses belong to the same <three parts>"

paths, as well as the twelve sources (that is, the six organs and six intestines), and the condition and inclination of each one, can be properly and definitely understood.

## CHAPTER SEVEN

*Whether any other pulse-locations are found in the three parts of the body besides those already mentioned which are suitable to investigate the twelve paths and their qualities*

When the Chinese lay out the whole human body into three parts (we have seen that in the previous chapter and the second,[110] to an extent[111]), they again explain each part of the body in the following way:

Text: The three parts of the body are the royal road for all liquids and solids; they are likewise the beginning and end of spirits.

Kipeus says: The three parts of the body are the source of suffering in man, as well as of temperaments.[112] Spirits arise from the substance of the vapors that the stomach accumulates; but the vapors go forth from the watery quality that resides in cavities, wherein they take their beginnings and ends.

Text: *Xám ciāo*, that is, the highest, or first part of the body, below the heart and chest, is located above the opening of the stomach. It governs the inner parts, not those which are carried out[113]. Its primary seat is the middle of the chest, below the location called *yo tam*—that is, the hall of jewels, at an interval of one finger-length and six parts. Simply put, where the nipples fall within,[114] the aforementioned part of the body ends.

*Chúm ciāo[115]*: that is, the middle or second part of the body, has its seat in that cavity of the stomach which is neither highest nor lowest. It governs flesh and nourishment. It is located on both sides of the navel.

---

[110] Could also be "in the previous chapter and after."

[111] *per transennam*, literally "through a net."

[112] *temperamentorum*, literally means "a mixture in due proportion." Exact meaning here unclear; "temperature"? "Temperament"? "Disposition"?

[113] *quae egeruntur*, literal translation, not sure what it refers to.

[114] *papillae interius incidunt*, literal meaning unclear.

[115] Could also be *"chúm ciao"* as the original text is unclear

Michal Boym

*Hia ciao*: that is, the lowest or third part of the body. It goes from the navel, descending to the highest opening of the ureters. It governs the location where pure substance is split off from the dregs, just as in regard to those things which are carried out. Its seat is below the navel, at one finger-measure. It also has a hall, which is the source and life of breath. Even when hot breaths intermingle by their own motion, they stick to everything, both inside and out. That motion is called the working inwards[116] of spirits.

Commentary: The seat of the highest part of the body is the middle of the chest, which is clear from the text. The seat of the middle part is on the side of the navel. The navel has two sides, but any given side has a location of a single finger-measure (where the belly hair covers the highest point), up to an interval of two finger-measures. In that location of radical wetness and primordial heat there is a pulse, as well as a path of fine, pure primordial heat from the meaning (meaning the stomach-path).

What food the stomach takes in, it processes and cooks, and first turns it into vapors, then into spirits, which come from the third part of the body and are carried to the twelve paths and stretch towards the routes or narrower passages, going up and down; or, these spirits, as though acting by force of their own heat, stir up the cavities of liquids and other <spirits>, and they permeate and disturb the blood. This motion, then, which the Spirits accomplish, runs from the location of the lowest, or third part. Although the original spirits take from elsewhere the substance of which they are at once constituted, yet because that very substance cannot exist without the spirits of the stomach, so too is it called their root and foundation. One must keep in mind that the hall and path of spirits lies in the third part of the body, where the motion of spirits begins and where all original spirits pass through due to that motion. So it happens that it is also called the root of the twelve paths, as well as the house and home of all twelve paths (which work their way into other spirits).

---

[116] *insinuatio*

26

*See the example in the previous chapter*

Therefore, in the same way that, in this universe, they create three particular units[117], called *Sān câi*, or very particular substantial virtues (that is, heaven above, earth below, and man himself in the middle, who partakes of both heaven and earth), so too do they divide the very body of man into three parts, like precincts: The Highest, which extends from the head to the opening of the belly and contains the lungs and chest, or whatever is above the diaphragm—the heart and pericardium, or, as they say, the wrapper of the heart; the Middle, which extends to the navel and encompasses the diaphragm, the stomach (or belly), along with whatever surrounds it, the spleen, and likewise the liver and gall bladder; and finally, the Lowest, which runs almost from the navel to the feet, and includes the kidneys, the bladder, the ureters, the intestines, and the slender intestines.[118] Otherwise, even the three previous regions are explained only with Metaphor, such that, in the highest part, they set something like various clouds; rain in the middle; and in the lowest, a lake and pools, which gathered from the aforementioned rain.

Then, they argue that three pulses in each hand correspond to these three sorts of regions of the human body in exactly the same way; and so, primordial heat governs the first and highest pulse (which they also indicate by the word for heaven, because it corresponds to the highest region of the body). Thus, this pulse is, by its own nature, overflowing, top-floating,[119] and great; radical wetness governs the Third or lowest pulse (which they indicate with the word for earth, because it corresponds to the lowest region in the body), and for that reason it is deep, and in comparison with the middle and highest pulse, is like a root, when a comparison is made with the trunk, branches, and leaves of a tree. They want this lowest pulse to be stronger in women,

---

[117] *tria... longe praecipua*, "three very particular things."

[118] *gracilia* <sc. *intestina*>. I think this is another name for the small intestines.

[119] *supernatans*

because radical wetness and blood predominate in them; but the highest pulse, that of the first region, is weaker in that sex. The opposite occurs with Men. But now, the middle pulse (which they indicate with the word for human, as this middle pulse, since it is between heaven and earth, corresponds likewise to the middle region of the body) is neither abundant nor deep, but gentler, they say (that is, moderate) and truly "middle," as one which shares in equal portion with both heat (which conducts itself to the first location) and with radical wetness (because it descends as though under its own weight to the earth and the lowest location). Likewise, it is called the boundary, as whatever is middle might limit the two extremes that we have discussed, no differently than the trunk of a tree does with its root and branches.

They do not only observe the aforementioned order of pulses, but they delve into each of them in an identical three-fold fashion. Thus, they first put a finger against someone's exterior, so that they only lightly press the skin; but when they approach the middle to examine it, they press down somewhat on the artery with their fingers. Finally, when they are going to examine the lowest region of the same pulse, something like the base or the root, they go for the very nerves and bones with a stronger touch, and in this way they surmise whether the same pulse exists everywhere; and thus, whether the disease is only superficial or is coming from the outside; or whether, on the other hand, because the inner parts are already engaged, it took root. Thus, if, as they are going to examine the base or root, they find that a pulse is missing, they faithfully proclaim that life has passed,[120] because (they say) the pulse is lacking a root. And since, at last, some of the organs are located on the left side of the human body, but others on the right; then they also show that <the latter>[121] organs tend towards the three pulses of the right hand, but <the former> tend towards the left-hand pulses.

---

[120] *actum esse de vita*, "it was done from life," idiom.

[121] *haec*, "this," can mean "the latter," where *ille*, "that," can mean "the former." It seems like that is what this author is doing here, but the Latin is

Table 3, Appendix, note 1

Thus, with regard to the pulses of those nine parts (namely, those that the three great regions of the body encompass), how they are found and how one's disposition[122] and qualities should be identified from the pulses, we shall explain below, with the addition of an example drawn by Chinese Doctors. Now, briefly:

Consideration[123] 1: Whatever pulse-locations will be found in the human body, for the purposes of determining wellness or diseases, life or death, one must use them to indicate the temperaments of those three regions of the body, and their inherent disposition, and whether they come on or presently sneak their way in.[124]

Consideration 2: That the pulse of any great region is divided into three parts each: be it top-floating (which comes from primordial heat), middling, or deep (which is in radical wetness); or, what amounts to the same, each one of the nine parts has its very own pulses.

Consideration 3: The character and affections of the exterior indicators or markers connected to those nine parts should be revealed by those pulses in the three parts of the pulses: that is, top-floating, etc., as has been already stated.

Consideration 4: Because *iam* and *in*, primordial heat and radical wetness, work themselves into the nine mentioned parts, it is necessary to determine the disposition of the pulses of one set of parts based on similar parts, and to illuminate the disposition of each individual part in the pulse of all parts. The reason is that

---

so strange and the topic so esoteric that I cannot be sure. He might just be translating something literally and clunkily from the Chinese. In this case, "the latter" would be organs on the right, "the former" would be organs on the left.

[122] *constitutio*

[123] *Collige*, literally, an imperative command, "Gather!" in the sense of "Understand this..."

[124] advenientes seu subinde irrepentes, exact nuance unclear. I think it is the difference between approaching head-on vs. moving in secretly.

any one will reveal not only its own disposition, but also how it interacts with other pulses with which it shares a certain sympathy or oneness. A further reason is that the paths between them are penetrated and mixed in a particular sort of way, from the one which is only proper to radical wetness, on to that which is meant only for primordial heat, and to another which takes its aqueous portion from each—again, the latter to the two previous ones, and the middle one of each part to that one which I mentioned in the first place, and to the last;[125] and so the pulse, which is called, one might say, "the path of the heart," reveals not only its own path to the heart, but even to the liver and bladder, and the paths to the lungs and stomach, and the things that are connected to these, along with the characters of each (as though by a subordinate token); and so it will be with the rest. For the three parts—heaven, man, and the earth, as they are called—contain each other jointly in the same way, for the part called heaven consists of the heaven-, man-, and earth-parts; and the part which is called earth again comes from heaven, man, and earth; and the part which is named man again arises from heaven, man, and earth. Likewise, that same part which contains the path of radical wetness is mixed with the paths that contain both radical wetness and primordial heat in equal measure, and are intersected by paths that contain only primordial heat; and that same part that contains the path of primordial heat is mixed with the paths that contain only radical wetness and with other paths that share equally in radical wetness and primordial heat. At the furthest point, that same part that contains the path possessing both radical wetness and primordial heat in equal measure, is shaped by the path that contains only primordial heat and by another path that contains only radical wetness. For that reason, the pulses that are found should not only mark out each path (each of the twelve indicating each one), but each pulse should indicate the paths, and all the individual pulse-paths,[126] not unlike with the source, and they should also indicate the things that form from them, the six fonts of life, in their own

---

[125] Meaning very unclear

[126] *omnes pulsus singular vias*, could also translate as "all the pulses <should indicate> each path.

disposition. So, for example, for the pulse-location which is called the paths of the heart, it is necessary for them to indicate not only their own path to the heart, but also the state and condition of[127] the liver and bladder, the lungs, the stomach, and the things connected to them. Then the pulse which is assigned to the location of the liver-path, indicates not only the disposition of the liver-path, but even of the heart and bladder, the stomach, the lunch, and the gate of life; and so on with the rest. But this is the cause of all these: life and wellness is something whole and entire, from which no one part of the body (although it may do so in a different way) or a single organ shares more in life than any other; and because all organs and intestines (the six fonts of life, as I call them) move in common towards the life and wellness of each part of the human body, and spread through the twelve paths in the blood and in the Spirits, which carry radical wetness and primordial heat.

Therefore, since life is an entire good, it cannot be life unless it comes from entire causes, and because evil comes from individual failings, then it is easy for life and wellness to fail from the least failing of a single organ or part, and so too each and every organ and intestine from which life emanates can easily be injured. Moreover, we will show below how, in one pulse which indicates the path of one organ, other paths can also reveal themselves and be determined—in other words, how, in one pulse in one part of the body, other parts of the body can reveal themselves and be determined.

In the meantime, we see that pulses of the twelve paths appear particularly in the hands, in which, thusly, there absolutely appears to be accumulation, like a gathering of pulses. For the topmost smaller part of the middle region of the body indicates the path of great radical wetness (the lungs) through a pulse in the right hand, and the smaller middle part of the middle region reveals the liver through the path of diminished radical wetness

---

[127] We enter into a series of genitives that could also go with *viam*: "not only the path to the heart (*via cordis*, lit. "path of the heart"), but also those to the liver...connected to them, their state and condition."

in the left hand; so it is absolutely said to be an accumulation, particularly in the hands. And although we just showed that the paths of the organs and intestines are found in the feet, yet because neither the pulses of all paths nor the chief ones have a foundation there, they should be looked for in the hands rather than in the feet. We shall pursue this, if we only look at it, whenever there are accumulations or gatherings in the human body: of the bones, marrow, sinews, organs and intestines, spirits, and finally veins and pulses; for if this last gathering of pulses should be found in the hands, it will be necessary to ascertain that locations in the hands are suitable for examining the twelve paths.

## CHAPTER EIGHT

*It is asked where in particular one may find the sources[128] of the things that the human body is made of; and whether pulses could be taken in each of them to understand the 12 paths, or whether such pulses exist only in the flowing of the veins, and whether they are different than in the hands.*

It is certain that the human body is made of bones, marrow, sinew, flesh, skin, blood, pulses, spirits, organs, and intestines; and so it is necessary to know the locations of the bones, marrow, nerves, etc., and to find their cognates. The Chinese place the kidneys in the first place, then the heart, followed by the liver and then the lungs, and next the spleen; but they say that the kidneys performs their actions in sixth place. Then, just as the kidneys start in the first location and so begin to perform their actions first of all; followed by the heart; the liver in the third place; next the lungs; and lastly the spleen. But these organs (just like the things that connect to the organs—that is, the intestines, the ureters, the small intestines, the gall bladder, the large intestines, and the stomach) and those remaining things have their own accumulation and locations, as can be seen in Table III (below).

Therefore, in the aforementioned location, *tu cau* (which refers to the great store[129]) is the source of the intestines.

In the location called *kí hŭ* (which refers to the steady union of qualities over the for seasons of the year) is the source of the six organs. Then, because the heart is not only the cause of the face and shoulders, but also the palms, hand, and also the tongue and

---

[128] *scaturigines*, an uncommon word that means "bubbling spring," used here (I believe) in the sense of "font" or "source" (like *fons* and *origo*).
[129] *magnum reconditorium*; *reconditorium* does not appear in Classical Latin (although it comes from a verb meaning "to hide away" or "to store away"). It does appear in later Latin, but not in a medical sense—one meaning is as a place where maps are stored, and the other is as a place where remains are stored (a mausoleum / crypt, I suppose).

blood, there is an accumulation of blood in the *kĕ yú* location, which refers to the location of the diaphragm.

The lungs, too, because they are not only the cause of the nose, lips, skin, hair, and nails, but also Spirits, are an accumulation of the spirits themselves in the *sān ciāo* location—that is, the three parts of the body.

Now the liver, because it is not only the source of the eyes but is also the font of the sinews, so the source of the sinews is in the *jaɱ lîm ciûen* location, which indicates the dwelling and source of heat.

The kidneys are not only the cause of the teeth and ears, but also of the bones. The source of the bones is in the *ta ín* location (which means great elevation). Likewise, the kidneys are the source too of marrow in the bones. The location where the source of the marrow lies is called *ciúe kŏ*, which means interruption of the bones.

There remains the accumulation and source of veins and pulses, which the Chinese say is able to exist nowhere else but the hands themselves, and they call *tá quên*, which means the abyss of great depth, and because, concerning the chief cause of veins and their origins, they teach that no organ, no intestine is the cause of the source,[130] they want the reader to understand that each and every organ and intestine runs together and is to a certain extent the cause of the origin of each vein.

Because no few paths to the aforementioned source-site of the veins flow from their sources (the organs and intestines) and come together; and because blood and spirits, as they move through the veins and their inherent Elementary qualities, will explain through these <qualities> the disposition both of the

---

[130] Throughout this passage, the author has used *cause* and *scaturigo* synonymously as "source," in reference to specific organs. *Causa* usually means "cause," but can be used as "original cause" or "source." *Scaturigo* means "bubbling-water" or "spring water," but just like *fons*, "spring," it means "source." This is the first time he's mixed the two together.

paths and the six fonts of life, they should produce a pulse by their own motion. Indeed, no pulse-location more appropriate could be found or chosen than where the veins meet up, for there too is a meeting of pulses.

Therefore, since this location is in the hands, the locations in the hands seem to be suitable for pulses; for looking into the twelve paths and their inherent Elementary qualities, as well as the origins from which the organs and intestines emanate. See table 3, notes 2, 3.

## CHAPTER NINE

*Why should pulses be looked for in the left hand, where the origin of the veins is found? Likewise, whether the left hand alone is sufficient, or whether pulses of veins should be looked for in the right hand as well?*

Practice dictates that pulses are found not only in the left hand, but also in the right one. The Chinese (as we have shown above), when they look for the sources of the things that make up the body, have said that the source of the veins is in the hands, and they declared it the source of pulses.

But in the right hand, the location called *ki keù*, mouth of spirits, they say also has pulses. Because this pulse in particular is created from the motion of spirits as they travel downward, they are convinced that an accumulation of pulses also exists in the right hand, and thus they decisively assert that the noblest pulse locations and their conjunctions[131] appear in either hand, and that there is sufficient reason in them as to why pulses should be sought not only in the left hand but the right, because although the origin of veins is in the left hand, motion in the veins arising from blood and Spirits creates a pulse.

Then, in the right-hand location called *ki keu*, because an accumulation of pulses is also found, they argue based on it that there is the greatest power and quantity of Spirits there, and necessarily, as they move down in the blood, they must produce motion at every point outside and inside the veins, and thus <produce> the pulse arising from this motion. Then they say that is very useful to check the pulses in both hands, because both the left and right hand have equal standing with pulses.[132] The left hand has blood flowing in the veins, where, of course, it is hidden and never appears in a living body without spirits; but the right hand has the supply of spirits, which, because they flow with blood, cannot exist without blood. Thus, because blood and

---

[131] *concursus*, translated also as "coming together" or "union," translated elsewhere as "meeting place."

[132] *causam adaequatam pulsuum*, literally, "an equalized cause of pulses."

spirits are the cause of motion and the motion of pulses, which are found in both the right and left hand, they had declared that the pulses can and should be taken at a location in both hands.

Consider too that some human organs and intestines are on the left, but others on the right; and so the paths flowing from them are some on the right, others on the left, as we have related above. Therefore, in order for their condition, and the condition of their inherent elemental qualities, to be understood, you must follow the pulses which are to be taken, in the left hand, according to left-hand organs and intestines; and in the right hand, according to the right-hand ones.

Finally, there is a very powerful reason that the pulse should be taken in the hands: because all that circulation of the blood and Spirits (which convey radical wetness and primordial heat, whence comes life) finally ends and is filled up in the hands, and from them again they start their circuitous course. Therefore, because the beginning of life and the end of life reveal themselves in the hands, they conclude with certainty that pulses should be taken nowhere else—although they reveal themselves also in the feet.

But it is necessary to explain how the circulation of the twelve paths in the human body, and the revolution in those <twelve paths> of the blood and the spirits that carry radical wetness and primordial heat, come to an end in the hands and begin from them as well, and thus how circulation is understood by the Chinese according to the pulses of the hands, and how it can be understood by anyone.

The circular shape and motion appears no more clearly in any other thing than in the celestial orbs, whose revolution,[133] which has been discovered by men based on their familiarity and long observation, is believed to be everlasting. But whether it can

---

[133] *circumvolutio*, "turning around." I do not know that the sciences had a clear understanding of the different between rotation and revolution, and so I will not observe a strict difference in the various words used here of turning.

exist from an eternal time, alongside creation or created things, is argued in the schools, and is confirmed by most Thomists.[134] Some say that the heavenly orb revolves in a span of twenty-four hours, and each year observes the circuit not only of the sun but of the other Planets as well; such a thing can be made everlasting by God. But some nations, taking Aristotle's lead, argue that it actually came from something everlasting.[135] Among the most learned of Philosophers and Mathematicians in our age and before, some deny that perpetual motion has been identified, others deny that it can been found, and others deny both of them, and rightly so.

But if constant motion can be granted, of course it must be said that it can be granted first to the heavenly spheres, then to the life of human bodies, and finally from artificial items, in clocks or tools which have their own motion, as in various subjects. No other figure easier or more fitting can be fashioned according to eternal motion than a circle, and in fact it describes it. The current motion of the heavens imitates it. Human life does as well, and so does his wheeled clock, a work of wondrous art, and the marvelous products of human skill.

It demonstrated supreme talent that a certain Painter was said to have drawn a completely perfect circle, flawlessly, without a compass. This too demonstrated supreme talent, that another Painter likewise showed that the center of the compass was eliminated with a single stroke;[136] in fact, that such progress was made by human effort that clocks were crafted, which come down and run about in the likeness of dogs, Lions, and human Characters at the hour; so that they successfully produced by

---

[134] *Thomism* is the philosophical school that arose as a legacy of the work and thought of Thomas Aquinas (1225–1274), philosopher, theologian, and Doctor of the Church. In philosophy, Aquinas' disputed questions and commentaries on Aristotle are perhaps his most well-known works.
[135] *de facto fuisse ab aeterno*, literally, "that it was in fact from the eternal."
[136] Meaning unclear

craft tools that ring of their own accord, with no encouragement, according to the numbers.

There recently appeared in Poland a clock which can show not only Lunar eclipses, but also the oppositions of Planets, their conjunctions; their fourth, sixth, and third aspects[137] (as is found at Prague and elsewhere), and the other monthly motions—even yearly ones. But what seemed particularly worthy of our admiration is that, with a single revolution of its wheels, it would illustrate most wonderfully the course of the stars, over six months, to each hour and day; sometimes even the course of the moon. You would say that it lived to the middle of the year. But whether or not something else could be achieved, to present a similar motion over a whole year seems eminently possible to me. In fact, it would not be ridiculous to believe that another would perhaps occur towards the end of the year, one which might bring forth a round instrument for motions for two or more years. Therefore, man's skillful investigation of external and circular things could compare[138] with lifeless tools, and for as long as half a year. But in truth, God, the Wisest Craftsman of all things, imposed a circular motion upon the enormous heavenly spheres, over vast span, thousands of years ago;[139] but because he also created living things in the world, akin to clocks,[140] who were granted various cycles of years, and ages, and bodies for the things that drew breath, most especially mankind. He wanted man to keep them as the foundations of life, and to guide them through the course of that life, and finally to meet their end within them, but in such a way that he granted eternal life in paradise to mankind through their use and consumption of the marvelous bounty that he bestowed, the staff of life.[141] Through this bounty, creeping into the body over a long duration, as it happens, the ravages of time (like a sort of

---

[137] *quadtratos, sextiles, et trinos aspectus*, meaning unclear.

[138] *conferre*, often means "compare," but the exact meaning here is a little unclear.

[139] *a tot annorum millibus*, literally, "from so many thousands of years."

[140] *quasi horologia*, literally, "as if a clock."

[141] *ligni vitae*, but the English phrase "staff of life" is used to refer to bread.

rust on the wheels of life) were uncovered. Not satisfied with this obviously divine generosity, he promised that same life in heaven, by far the most perfect and abounding in all good things, if only (as is fair) one obeyed the will of their most holy Creator. Therefore, since a circular motion is in complete accordance with our life (because, of course, it is primarily compared with that),[142] we must believe that a circular motion in living things, and especially in man, is most appropriate.[143]

Thus, the Chinese frequently argue that not only should human life should be measured by the motions of the heavens, but that it is in fact very similar to them. Indeed, we Europeans count our lives by yearly circular motions; but the Chinese have revealed yearly and monthly circular motions in the human body, and even long-lasting ones (which have been around almost since the flood).[144]

We shall now demonstrate how they came to understand this, following their teaching, the origin of long-lasting circular motion, which is inherent in our lives, and likewise the place where it begins and where it ends. But then we shall attempt to explain the monthly cycle of our life, even until our last year, GOD willing.

The Chinese propose to place the center of a circle (such as you may describe with a compass) in a plane, and the beginning of an orb at some point on a flat surface, but to join the end of the perpetual orb at its oblique bend, and so, day after day, to travel back and forth from the point that it began;[145] and if motion, once undertaken and completed, persists in that plane, it again will return whence it came and accordingly will produce a variety of circular motions and follow them through. They constantly assert that it happens in quite the same way in the human body.

---

[142] *quod quippe quo maxime conferatur*, exact meaning unclear

[143] *maxime regularem*, with the sense of "most in accordance with the rules."

[144] *jam inde ab ipso prope diluvio*, "already then from nearly the flood itself."

[145] Literal translation; maybe describing a Chinese compass?

It is beyond doubt, they say, that life begins when the fetus is endowed with breath,[146] but the lifecycle is longer for some people, shorter for others, and that because the vital circle of a long life has a thicker circumference, but that of a short life is narrower. They want some vital circles to be contained by this circle, and others to be inserted in them in turn, much as the globe is formed from yearly circles, lunar (or monthly) circles, and daily ones. If the circle of life has begun, it should have a place from which it began, and one towards which it flows in its course and comes to an end, to restart its course again, just as the heavenly orbs move from a starting point until they again set of from the same starting point.

But what exactly, we ask, is the center of this vital circle in the human body? The Chinese say that it is the middle part of the human body. But what is its circumference?[147] They say it's the head, the feet, and the hands. But if you set the foot in the middle of the circle, as though it were a point in the human body, and trace around it with the other foot, it describes a perfect circle, to the distance of the feed, head, and hands. And so, since life exists in this entire span and circuit based on the actual motion of the parts which touch the circumference, it necessarily touches the circular circumference from the motion of the parts and describes it. Then, having shown the center and periphery of the circle, we must show how the twelve paths are assigned through it, from the center and around the center; and how blood and spirits are assigned through them; and finally, how radical wetness and primordial heat are assigned in them in their own vehicles (that is, how the life resulting from them is borne); or rather, finally, how that flow of life goes from the center to the circumference, from where motion takes its start in this vital wheel and uses up the course of life.

---

[146] *animatur*, "make animate," "give breath," "give a soul to." *Anima* in Latin is literally the breath of life, and is used interchangeably. Most often in this book, *anima* and its related words will be translated as "soul," since the term specifically used of the process of breathing here is *spiratio*.
[147] *circumferentia*

41

Michal Boym

*But let us hear from the Chinese themselves*

Text: A person takes Spirits from food; food is taken into the stomach and shares its virtues with the five organs and six intestines, for everything that is in the body takes Spirits, which come from the substance of the food; for that which is subtle is *qûm*, wet, that is, the purest blood, endowed with radical wetness, as it creeps through the veins. That which is thick and not yet well-digested is *quêi*, something like a mass of hot spirits that are endowed with primordial heat, travelling inside and outside the veins and carrying blood. Of course, these two things, *qûm* and *quêi*, penetrate and surround the whole body, like a wheel or a circle, which travels around without interruption. Note: this is because hot spirits are subject to primordial heat, and the blood in the veins is subject to radical wetness, and these two things, mixed and suffused with each other, perform their circular motion in the human body in the span of twenty-four hours; in that span of time, 50 heavenly homes[148] are travelled, using the Chinese expression; and in the same span of time, the Spirits and blood which started their course from the path of the lungs early the previous day (the third or fourth hour in Europe, for each Chinese hours takes two European hours) flow back and forth for a whole day and a whole night, and they finish their whole course there, in the very place where the greatest mass of spirits is found (which is called the mouth of Spirits) and where primordial heat and radical wetness appear, joined to each other by turns, and from where these things begin to flow back and forth again in the blood and Spirits, and form permanent orbs,[149] and carry life about in them.

Text: As for the pulses of the twelve paths and the pulses of the fifteen *lŏ* veins (these are pulses in the veins that trickle like streams[150] to the sides of the twelve paths), where do they take their beginning, and where do they end? Blood and Spirits flow

---

[148] *domus coelorum*, literally "homes of the skies." It seems that this is a measure of angle, in the same way we use degrees, minutes, and seconds.
[149] *perpetuos orbes*, maybe another term for circulation?
[150] *rivulos*, literally, "small brooks," diminutive form of *rivus*, "stream," "brook."

down in the twelve pulse-paths, they intersect and are intersected by radical wetness and primordial heat, so that they invigorate, support, maintain, and give life to the entire human body. Their source (that is, the source of the blood and spirits) is in the middle, or rather, the center part of the middle region of the body (which we have said is above the center of the vital circle); but then, once they are shared, they trigger the motion of the path of great radical wetness for the hands from that source, and go on to the path of bright (pure) primordial heat in the hands, and from there to the path of pure and bright primordial heat for the feet, and from there to the path of great radical wetness for the feet; from there then, they continue on to the path of diminished radical wetness for the hands, and from there to the path of great primordial heat for the hands, and then from there to the path of great heat for the feet, and then to the path of diminished radical wetness for the feet. It follows the same motion on to the path of defective radical wetness for the hands, and from there to the path of diminished heat for the hands, and at last, from there to the path of defective radical wetness for the feet; where, of course, that vital wheel of blood and spirits, and the circuit, ends. Turning around then, it returns from the site of the path of great radical wetness, and so forth, by the course which we have repeatedly described.

The motions of the paths that we discussed, being exactly like rings or interlocking circles, intersect with one another and travel around the entire body without interruption, but in the morning, they return to their location in the right hand and then being to flow and course again. So it is that a judgment can be made on any sort of disease, even on life and death itself, based on this location in the hands (which is also called the mouth of spirits).

You may observe here, almost in glimpses,[151] that because there are fifteen *lŏ* (routes or paths) rising up at the sides of the paths,

---

[151] *quasi per transennam*, literally, "as if through a net / lattice."

they create various path as well by three different movements and pulses, as shall be discussed below.

Each day, at an early hour (*ym*), which is the third or fourth European hour of the morning, a motion and bending begins to take place, for it starts in the center of the large part of the body, and is shared with the lungs; hence, the motion of blood and spirits starts with the lungs, and courses down from there to the large intestines; from there, though, it goes to the stomach, from the stomach to the spleen, and then to the heart, and then to the small intestines, and from there to the ureters and the bladder, or kidneys; from the bladder or kidneys to the wrapper of the heart, and then to the lowest, or third region of the body, and then to the gall bladder, and finally to the liver. This motion concludes in the same place in the first and second hours of the night. In the third and fourth hours of the following day, it once again resumes its course to the lungs, and so, following this course for the subsequent days, months, and years, it completes its own proper measure of life. Therefore, because the head and foundation of all paths is found in the lungs, or rather, in the path of the lungs; that is, when blood runs through them (and again, blood and the motion of blood is no different than the spirits that the lungs hold sway over), and since the course from the aforementioned location takes place during the morning hours, the pulse in the veins should also begin from that same place; it comes about that the pulses in the right-hand location must be examined.

Text: Once you know the beginning and end, it is easy to determine how radical wetness and primordial heat are situated. Why do we say this?[152] Because, of course, the end and beginning of pulses, and furthermore, of radical wetness and primordial heat, are the seat from which they begin to move in the morning like a wheel. So we have said that the beginning is set there, but the end is also set there, in fact, because obviously the spirits of the three paths of radical wetness take their end from <the spirits> of the three paths of primordial heat; when

---

[152] *Quare hoc dicitur*, literally, "For what reason is this said?"

they end, death follows. But the individual paths of such a death have their own markers, and so we say that they have an end.

Commentary: Each individual thing has its own heat within it, and its own wetness, and thus their end and beginning is found in those heat- and wetness-locations that were already determined. Then, in the pulse-paths, there are two important bonds[153]; as well as in this aforementioned location, *ki keu*, because the pulses of the three paths of radical wetness and the three of primordial heat are seen there in the right hand early in the morning, and they begin to move and circulate.[154] Therefore, the motion's beginning comes from the spirits and primordial heat; but that is the end and terminal point for the pulse, and then for the three paths of radical wetness and the three paths of primordial heat. But it is called the end, because radical wetness finds its end.

What follows are the signs of death in anyone. First, the signs of failing[155] Spirits of diminished radical wetness for the bladder or kidneys[156] are sharp and protruding teeth, and a withering and dryness of the flesh. Second, the signs of failing spirits of radical wetness for the stomach <and> the feet are: swelling of the body, and a twisting of the lips away from each other at an angle. Third: the signs of failing Spirits of defective radical wetness for the liver are: the tongue swelling into a round shape. Fourth: the signs of failing Spirits of great radical wetness for the lungs are: dryness of the skin and body, and likewise a loss or stiffening of the head- and body-hair.[157] Fifth: the signs of failing Spirits of

---

[153] *vincula*, literally, "chains," "manacles," "fetters." In some way showing things are bound together.

[154] *circulari*, "to go In a circle"

[155] *desinentium*, literally, "ceasing"

[156] *Vesicae seu renum humidi radicalis diminuti, Spirituum desinentium signa sunt*, a string of genitives whose relationship isn't entirely clear to me. I'm assuming that the "radical wetness" possess the "failing / ending Spirits", all of which belong to the "bladder or kidneys." The remaining several signs of death follow a similar pattern, and I'll translate them accordingly.

[157] *capillorum ac crinium*

lessened radical wetness for the heart are: teeth that appear deep black. Next, a sign of failing spirits of primordial heat in the three paths for the eyes are vision loss,[158] almost as though shadows were gradually pouring over them. Finally, the signs of failing spirits of primordial heat for the six paths lie in cold sweat, which appears like jewels and does not flow over the rest of the body, and indicates an immediate exhaustion of spirits, followed by death. Therefore, whoever witnesses these indications, do not doubt that death is certain.

It follows[159] from what has been said that: 1) pulses must be taken not only in the left hand, where there is the greatest accumulation both of veins and blood (in which the pulses form), but pulses must also be taken in the right hand, where, in the identical *ki keŭ* location, there is a great strength and quantity of spirits, which flow in the blood in a living person and move it as well, from which motion pulses arise. In fact, the pulse should first be taken in this right-hand location because the wheel of life (that is, the circulation[160] of blood and spirits, as discussed above) find their beginning and end in that same place.

It follows that: 2) life in man (that is, radical wetness and primordial heat) is shared with the whole body for no other reason than that the same life extends from the center (which is in the central region of the body) to the edge of the hands, head, and feet; with the help of the motion of blood and spirit, it travels within and through the whole body, in a circle, like some sort of wheel; it travels and turns from the location and path of the lungs, taking its own course. Continuing on the same course in a perfect circle for a natural day (this is, twenty-four European

---

[158] *obscuratio illorum*, literally, "a dimming of those things <the eyes>," I think this refers to an inability to see rather than a change in the color of the eyes.

[159] *Colligitur*, literally, "it is gathered together." I translate this throughout at "it follows."

[160] *circuli*, literally, "circles." The text only uses *circulatio* once (I believe), but any instances in my translation of "circulation" are renderings of Latin words that relate to the word "circle." I have followed a similar tack with words like *gyrus*, *circuitus*, and *cyclus*.

hours), and by comparing not only the cycles of daily motion, but also monthly and yearly, it arrives at the appropriate period or endpoint that fits its own causes, <or however else it carries other things>[161]; and this endpoint is called Death.

But how have the Chinese come to understand that the circular motion of blood and Spirits start from the lungs and their path, <and that too> because pulses start in the right-hand location in the morning? The answer is: life begins with breathing (which comes from inhalation—that is, the drawing in of air—and exhalation[162]—that is, the ejection of air; and these two things are called systole and diastole[163]). Therefore, because the lungs are the workshop of breathing, and because life (as we have said) begins with breathing and ends when it ends, it clearly follows from what has been said that life begins in the lungs themselves, and again ends in the lungs; that is, blood and Spirits (which are the vehicles of life) begin the circulation of life in the path of the lungs, and they return to the same path, only to start there again.

It also follows that the motion of life and pulses (through which life reveals itself, since the path of the lungs ends in that place), both exists and is obvious in the right-hand location, which is called *ki kĕu*, the mouth of spirits, and is without a doubt the endpoint of the path of the lungs (which are the workshop of spirits, since they create pulse and motion by their own heat).

But what will you say is the cause for the lung-path ending in the right-hand location? What cause, I say, for the mass, force, and supply of spirits being there? Why does the pulse start there in the morning, and why must it be taken in the morning in order to properly detect a sickness in the system? All of these things will become clear in the next chapter, where again we shall deal

---

[161] Also could be "although something brings it." Exact meaning unclear.

[162] *introspiratio* and *exspiratio*, literally, "breathing in" and "breathing out."

[163] *systole* and *diastole*, from the Greek συστολή, meaning "drawing together" or "contraction," and διαστολή, meaning "drawing apart" or "separation."

Michal Boym

with the measure of time and the motion of pulses and of circulation.[164]

## CHAPTER TEN

*Why it is best for pulses to be taken in the morning, and likewise, where and how many pulse-locations there are in each hand.*

Text: The Emperor Huanti offers the following sort of question: For one who takes pulses, why is it best to be done in the morning? Kipeus answers: Because in the morning, the spirits of radical wetness are not yet disturbed by great agitation, nor are the spirits of primordial heat dispersed; likewise, food and drink have not yet been taken into the body, nor have the pulse-paths yet been refilled; the vein streams[165] similarly still observe the pulse; and lastly, the blood and spirits have not yet been disturbed. Thus, this time is suitable above all others to take pulses.

Text: Behind the palm of the hand is a sort of bone that sticks out a little bit, whose name is the boundary.[166]

Commentary: If you draw a straight line from the thumbnail directly behind the joint,[167] which is between the arm and the hands, there exists a bone that sticks out a little bit; this is the arm's pulse (called the *quan*), which must be kept well in mind. Behind the palm, there exists the sublime mouth, immediately under which one may find the pulse-location (which is called the boundary).

Text: In order (from this location), note and set in order the location *chě* which indicates the Chinese cubit (and is much smaller than Europe's), and you will note carefully three locations or points.

Commentary: Whenever you take a pulse, before anything else, you should place the middle finger of the hand, which is the third from the thumb, below the location of that bone that sticks out somewhat, and in this way, you will have determined the seat of

---

[165] *venarum rivuli*
[166] *limes*, literally, "cross-path," but comes to mean "limit" or "boundary" ("dividing line")
[167] *juncturam & flexum*, "the connection and bending."

that pulse's point, which is called *quañ* or boundary. Going straight ahead through the pointer finger, touch the point call *cuñ pú*; and the third finger, which follows the middle finger and is called the 'ring-finger',[168] will fall upon the third point of the pulse called *chĕ pù*.

Text: Travelling from the aforementioned location in the palm of the hands, *iuci*, up the protruding bone (*quañ*), there is a distance of one finger-joint[169]; but by traveling half this distance,[170] from this point (*quun*) to the elbow (*chĕ cĕ*), which indicates a gap of a cubit. Between the two points thus assigned, one finds a middling location or point, which is in front of the *cuñ* and behind *chĕ*, often called the *quañ* location (that is, the boundary), because primordial heat, with the aid of spirits, goes out towards *cuñ*, the first location. Radical wetness, with the help of blood in veins, returns towards *chĕ*, the third location; thus it happens that the distinct paths of threefold primordial heat (as the heat departs) end at that location, like at a border; and the same number of paths of threefold radical wetness end there too when the wetness returns. For this reason, one sees a threefold motion of primordial heat and a threefold <motion> of radical wetness.

The motion of spirits (which come from primordial heat) proceeds from the third location (*chĕ*) and the second location (*quañ*) and advances to the first location, which is called *c'um̄*. The motion of blood, though, which comes from radical wetness, emanating from the first location *c'uñ*, advances through the second location *quan* up to the third location, called *chĕ*.

From the first pulse-location, called *c'um̄*, one learns of the constitution of the topmost part of the body, which runs from the top of the head to the breast, and extends as well to the skin of the body and the hair. In the second pulse-location, one learns of the constitution of the middle part of the body, which runs from

---

[168] *annularis <digitus>*, literally, "<the finger> of the ring."
[169] *articuli*, "joint" or "knuckle." Again, the exact measurement is uncertain
[170] *medium ...illius spatii*, literally, "the middle / half of that extent."

the chest to the navel and encompasses everything contained therein. In the third pulse-location, one learns of the constitution of the lowest part of the body, which runs from the bottom-most part of the stomach to the soles of the feet.

From these, it follows that there are three locations or points in each of the right and left hands, and in those points, a Physician should take the pulse likewise with three fingers.

Secondly, it follows that the middle or second pulse-location in the right hand is obviously where the mouth of spirits is, and in the left hand, the middle and second pulse location is where the confluence of veins, called the *tai quên*, or by another name, *gîn im*, the crossroads of man; that is, the intersection of primordial heat and radical wetness.

But why have the names limit and Chinese cubit been given to this pulse-location? I shall reveal a secret: Chinese doctors believe that vein courses, through which blood and spirits come and go, if they were extended and someone wanted to measure their length, would contain 810 (*cham*[171]), meaning it in such a way that the spirit, always maintaining its proportion, contains a measure between even the body itself, insofar as it is larger or smaller. There is, then, a Chinese measure *cham*, which measures twice the distance between both arms; and this is agreed to consist of 10 other smaller measure, the aforementioned *chĕ* (which is the word used for the Chinese cubit, which is smaller than the European cubit). *Chĕ*, then, is made up of ten finger-measures, called *cuñ*. Therefore, if we wish to make the aforementioned distance of the veins, running from the furthest part of its middle finger, it is 810 *chăm*, beginning from the first measure of *cham*; that is, those smaller measures that it contains occur—namely, *chĕ* and *cùn*. So it follows that the first cubit-measure *chĕ*, up to the forearm, ends in the third pulse-location that we assigned previous and called *chĕ*, for the *cùn* measure (that is, the finger-joint) loses its name

---

[171] In the text Cham has a bar over the m. For typesetting purposes in this text the bar is being placed over the 'a'.

in that location—for instance, the path of primordial heat, through the overflowing pulse (*feu*), which one senses by a light touch on the surface of the skin and flesh; but it is detected by radical wetness, which have gas it through the deep pulse *Xin*, from a rather strong touch against the bones.[172] The second, or middle location, which shares equally in heat and wetness, is found through the *huōn* pulse; that is, the remiss pulse, the one that is neither floating nor deep. For this reason, when taking the pulse *in cuṁ* and *in chĕ*[173], one covers almost that whole area with three fingers, but with this distinction: of course, the first finger will take on the *yâm*, or primordial heat, as it is touching the first location; and the third finger, as it is touching the third location, will take *yñ*; that is, radical wetness. But the large, or middle finger, touching the location in a prime position to take a pulse,[174] will differentiate between *yâm* and *iñ* at a single touch.

Text: Pulses of veins have the *chĕ* and *c'uṁ* location. Why? Because, *chĕ* and *c'un* contain the substance of fundamental elements;[175] it holds dominion over radical wetness in the middle location *quān* up to *chĕ*, so that one should distinguish that the *cuñ* joint marks the same *chĕ* location; likewise, one should distinguish *chĕ*, and compare it with the *cuñ* location, wherein mastery of primordial heat lies.

Commentary: Pulses have three locations in the organs: *cuñ*, *quān*, and *chĕ*. The *quān* location is in the middle, where, if you continue on to the *yn ci* cavity, you have a distance of *cuñ* (that is, the measure of a finger-joint). This span then is subject[176] to the primordial heat as it departs the limit (that is, the *quān* location). But if you continue on from the *quān* limit to the *chĕ*

---

[172] Meaning and grammar unclear.

[173] Not sure if *in* is Chinese, or a Latin preposition: "in *cum* and in *che*"

[174] *exploratissime*, literally, "Most exploredly;" this is the verb used of taking a pulse, so I think it's just emphasizing that the middle finger is in a very good position for that.

[175] *principalium rerum congeries*, "heaps of first things."

[176] *subicitur*, literally, "it is cast under," I have translated it with the cognate "subject."

*cě* location, it measures the span of *chě*, the Chinese cubit, and it acquires its name, and this span is subject to returning radical wetness.

From this, it is understood that radical wetness occupies the space of a tenth of a finger-joint, within the measure of *chě*, or the Chinese cubit (the beginning of which you should take from the tip of the ring finger). But the primordial heat residing within *cun* (meaning that finger-joint which is ninth, counting from the tip of the middle finger) occupies only nine parts of that *cun* (see below). Thus, *chě* and *cun* are the beginning and end of pulses—that is, one joint, which is called *chě* and nine parts of the other joint; thus, those locations are called *cun* and *chě*.

Commentary: Note, each measure *cun* has 10 completely equal parts; and the final measure of *cun* (that is, the tenth measure of the finger joints, which add up to *chě*, the Chinese cubit), is a whole joint. The radical wetness residing in that span, occupying an even[177] and equal number of equal parts, is most perfect (and it is called *lúo in*); that is, mature and most perfect wetness. An odd number is found (granted it still contains equal parts, but in an odd number, in the ninth part of the joint), which we call *quān cǔn* and is the first pulse-location), for the tenth equal part, tending towards an even number and the complete joint,[178] enters the palm of the hand, as you can see in the figure. Thus, in the aforementioned *cuñ* joint's odd number, primordial heat claims only nine parts, and in them *lao yân* holds sway, which, when mature and most perfect, indicates primordial heat.

And so, just as an even number is given to radical wetness, so too is an odd number given to primordial heat. Therefore, within the Chinese cubit *chě*, one must distinguish radical wetness and primordial heat, as well as those locations that they occupy—*chě*, of course, or rather, its whole finger-joint, which completes

---

[177] *par*, meaning literally "equal," "like," or "fair," here I believe refers to types of number: "even." I will translate it accordingly; by that same token, I have translated *impar*, its opposite, as "odd."
[178] *integritatem articuli*, "the wholeness of the joint," exact meaning unclear.

Michal Boym

that measure and is in the tenth number, counting from the tip of the middle finger, and the nine parts of the *cuñ* joint, which are the two foundations and boundaries of pulses, as well as the noblest locations of the veins, where health, illnesses, and whatever damages health are revealed all at the same time; and so, knowledge of all these things should be acquired.

## CHAPTER ELEVEN

*What fonts of life the three pulse locations (found both in the right and left hand) reveal the status and condition of, and what their[179] internal order is while doing so.[180] Likewise, it is explained what the reason is for that order, as well as what the reason is for its lightness and heaviness,[181] which is added to the pulses.*

Text: The pulses indicating the condition of the heart come from the path of lessened radical wetness to the hands, which begins from the heart itself; for the other path, which reveals the condition of the small intestines, it is the path of great primordial heat in the hands. These, I say, are the pulses in the first location of the left hand, called *cuñ kiū*, behind the *quan* location. Both paths join in the uppermost part of the body at the hall of spirits in the *quey ici* location, that is, the tail of the turtle.

The pulses indicating the condition of the liver are detected in the middle location (called *quan*) of the left hand; and <those indicating> the condition of the path which is called *cò kiue yñ kīm* (that is, the path of defective radical wetness from the feet to the head); and likewise for the further path that reveals the condition of the gall bladder and is called *ho xaō yam kīm* (that is, the path of diminished heat to the feet). These pulses, I say, are found in the second location (called *quān*) of the left hand. Both paths join in the middle region of the body, in the location called *pao muen*, which means the gate of membranes.[182]

The pulses indicating the condition of the bladder or kidneys are detected in the third location of the left hand, in the path of lessened radical wetness going from the feet. The ureters, however, whose condition is taken in the same way, are found

---

[179] Here, in reference to the pulse-locations.
[180] Literally, "in what order they reveal <the status and condition> amongst themselves."
[181] *levitatis et gravitatis*, a literal translation.
[182] *portam membranarum*

in the path of great heat going to the feet. Both paths unite in the lowest part of the body, which is called *quān yuên cò*, that is, "the seat of the source of clauses."[183]

The pulses indicating the condition of the lungs, and the condition of the path that runs from them, is called *Xeú tai yn kim*, that is, the path to the hands of great radical wetness. Likewise, for the other path that leads from the large intestines and is called *Xeu jam mim*, that is, the path from the hands of pure and bright primordial heat. Moreover, these pulses are found in the first location of the right hand, behind the *quan* location; but both paths unite in the location in the first part of the body called *hu kiě chi fu*; that is, the city of exhalation and inhalation, in the determined point that is called *yuén muěn*; that is, the gate of clouds.

The pulses indicating the condition of the spleen come from the path from the feet of great radical wetness and are found in the second location of the right hand. An identical process occurs there for another path, that is, the pulse of the stomach from the path of pure primordial heat to the feet. Both those paths intersect each other and come together in *chum ciao*, that is, the middle region of the body (also called the center[184]), which lies between the spleen and the stomach.

The pulses indicating the condition of the gate of life and the path that runs from it are called the path of defective radical wetness to the hands. But for the other path that reveals the condition of the third part of the body and is called the path of diminished heat from the hands, the pulses are found in the third location of the right hand, called *chě*. Both these paths intersect and come together in the lowest region of the body.

It follows that the pulses which are detected in the first location of the left hand indicate the condition of the heart and the small

---

[183] *clausarum originumsedes*, I translated *originumsedes* as two words: *originum sedes*.
[184] *meditullium*, literally equivalent to "middle earth," but meaning more the interior of a country, and thus the center or middle generally.

intestines, the dispositions of their paths, and furthermore, the situation of the uppermost part of the body. And so, it follows for the rest.

But why is it that, in the three aforementioned pulse-location, both in the right and left hands, Chinese doctors teach that the twelve paths and their sources (the things from which they came), as well as their disposition, can be detected in the aforementioned order? It will be beneficial to answer that from the locations[185] themselves.

Text: The pulse has three locations, and each location has four paths: that is, the path of great radical wetness for the hands and of bright primordial heat for the feet; likewise, that of great primordial heat and of diminished radical wetness for the feet. For this reason, in the pulse-locations, some of the paths extend this way, some that; others are marked from the first pulse-location, others from the third.

Commentary: Three pulse-locations exist in both the left and right hands. Each one indicates two paths, and thus the same location (for instance, the first in each hand) indicates four paths; and so it follows for the rest.

From the organs we have mentioned many times now, the lungs and their paths are in the uppermost location of the human body; but the bladder or kidneys in the lowermost. Thus, in the right hand (because the lungs[186] reside in the right-hand part of the uppermost part of the body), the lungs and their path (that of great radical wetness in the hands) are situated in the uppermost and first pulse-location, just as it is with the attached large intestines and their path, which is the path of bright primordial heat for the hands. Both paths are subordinate to the Element of Metal (in the opinion of the Chinese), which also produce top-

---

[185] *illis ipsis*, literally, "from those very things." It seems like it must be referring to the pulse-paths here.

[186] *membrum pulmonum*, literally, "the organ of the lungs." The author uses this strange expression frequently.

floating pulses because of the quantity of spirits; and these pulses indicate their condition in the first location.

Next, the kidneys or bladder, and their path (that of diminished radical wetness for the feet); and the ureters and their path, which is the path of great primordial heat for the feet, points to the left in the lowest part of the both; and both, because they are subject to the Element of water (whose nature is to flow to the lowest level) find the pulses that indicate their disposition in the lowest, or third pulse location in the left hand.

Text: The paths of radical wetness and primordial heat for the hands point towards the (Chinese) Element of Metals.

The paths of radical wetness and great primordial heat for the feet point towards the Element of water (they say that the Chinese produce water from the Element of Metals) which always seeks lower ground and cannot climb, and so the pulse of the path of the bladder (kidneys) and ureters stays in the lowest and last location in the hands.

The paths of defective radical wetness and diminished primordial heat point towards the Element of the trees, or rather, that of air; and they produce in the hands the fiery paths of great primordial heat and diminished radical wetness, for because the substance of the element of fire goes up and cannot move down, it happens that even the paths of the heart achieve a higher pulse location, especially on the left, where the heart resides. Because the path of fire produces the paths of great radical wetness and bright heat for the feet (which paths proceed from the earthen spleen and stomach), and because the location of the Element of earth is in the middle, so those paths in the spleen and stomach occupy the middle pulse (that is, the second location) in the right hand.

All five elements, and the things that they rule over, are placed in the order that they produce themselves. This is true for organs, intestines, and their paths, which have the virtues of the Elements and take their name from them.

Commentary: The lungs and large intestines of a metallic nature produce water—or rather, the kidneys and the ureters, which have watery properties. Thus, because the lungs are an organ on the right, and because they hold the location of the great highest part above the heart, their pulse also reveals the dispositions in the first location in the right hand.

But because the bladders (kidneys), together with the ureters, are on the left, in the large lowest part of the body, and because the water that holds power over them seeks the lowest point as it flows, their paths hold the last pulse in the left hand—that is, the pulse of the sixth location. And because water (the bladder) is the mother of trees and air (that is, those that indicate the condition of the liver and gall bladder in the left hand, over the bladder-location), they occupy the second or middle location (because they are also in the left part of the large region). But just as trees produce wood and air produces fire (which seeks higher levels), the heart and small intestines and their paths point to the Element of fire, and are in the left-hand part of the topmost region.

And so, the pulses that indicate their constitution occupy the first location in the left hand; but because fire is the producer of ashes and earth (which resides in the middle), it also points to the middle part of the body. Likewise, the spleen (which tends towards the right, along with the stomach; and which is given the name of "earth") points to the middle part of the body. As for the pulses that indicate the affections of the paths of the spleen and stomach, they have their seat in the middle or second location of the right hand. Finally, although the gate of life has fiery qualities, yet its nature is watery. For this reason, it is often called by the name bladder or kidneys, and its spirits consist of watery vapors, whose seat is there. Thus, the gate of life has taken the lowest, or third location in the right hand, and the pulses that indicate its[187] path, just as the paths of the third part of the body, which are connected to the aforementioned gate. In

---

[187] *suam*, grammatically should refer to the "gate of life's" path, but could refer to the pulse: "the pulses that indicate their own paths"

this manner, they have taken six locations, both in the left and right hand, according to the order of the Elements, the twelve paths, and their pulses. Thus, in short, you should follow this order: the pulses of the twelve paths begin, of course, in the first location of the right hand, which comes from the path of metallic lungs and from the path of the large intestines. These paths produce the paths of the watery bladder (the kidneys and ureters) in the last location of the left hand. These, then, produce the paths of the airy or tree-like liver and gall-bladder, in the middle location of the left hand. These, then produce the paths of the heart and small intestines in the first location of the left hand; and these paths, which were said to be very nearby in the third location of the right hand (because they have fiery qualities that complement each other), together with the paths of the heart and the small intestines, produce the paths of the gate of life and the third part of the body. But the fiery paths produce in the nearby middle location earth and ash, the nature of which is shared by the spleen and the stomach; thus, the paths of those things, even those that are called pulses because of them,[188] situated in this location as well. Even when the spleen and stomach (that is, earth) produce metals, whose nature is shared by the lungs and large intestines, the paths for both are found in the first location of the right hand. And so forth.

It follows that the lower pulse-paths for the organs and intestines have the lowest (that is, third) location; and the uppermost paths have the upper location, and the middle paths the middle location. But because those that have the higher ground are light, and those that hold the lower ground are thought to be heavy, we must ask whether the lightness and heaviness of a substance are found in the pulses according to the aforementioned shared order.[189]

The Chinese, after they had observed in the shared order of the universe that those Elements that held the uppermost location are least heavy, but those that held the lower location are most

---

[188] Exact meaning unclear.

[189] *coordinationem*, "coordination"

heavy, and those that held the middle location are less heavy, or partly-light and partly-heavy, and that there are also certain organs in the human body (which they also call Elements) that are in the uppermost part, and that the pulses indicating their paths hold that location in both the left and right hand. <After all that>, they persuaded themselves that the pulses in that first location should be the least heavy; but the lowest pulses (those of the lower organs) were the heaviest. Finally, those that were detected in the middle location were less heavy, or rather, partly-light, partly-heavy.

Text: Why do pulses have heaviness and lightness? An answer: The pulse in the highest location has a weight of the three small beans,[190] and its condition is detected on the surface of the skin and its connected hairs, and it indicates the path of the lungs. But if you should see that a pulse has the weight of six beans, and then that it is detected in the compression of veins and blood, you will understand that this is a heart-pulse. But if you take a pulse of nine beans, and that with a stronger touch to the flesh, that is a stomach-pulse, in the middle location. But if there is a weight of twelve beans and the pulse is taken by touching the sinews,[191] that is the liver-pulse, in the middle location.

Then, whatever pulse is found by putting the hand to the bones themselves, that will be the bladder's pulse (which is also called the gate of life) and will have a weight of fifteen beans. Therefore, it should be said that heaviness and lightness reside in pulses according to their shared order, which have been shared between the locations of the organs and intestines, and by the paths that proceed from them.

Commentary: A light[192] thing is subtle, floating at the surface, clearly very much like the heavens; a heavy[193] thing is dense, tending towards the deep, most like earth, because it shares in both. The five organs have heaviness; they also have lightness;

---

[190] *parvarum fabarum*, not sure what the converts to in modern units.
[191] *in attactu nervorum*, "in / at the touch of nerves / muscles."
[192] *leve*
[193] *grave*

some are located here, others there. Their spirits tend sometimes towards the surface, other times deep, since they have a similarity with the heavens and earth. Thus, based on the various pulses in lightness and heaviness, we find the order of heaviness and lightness that follows. The wings of the lungs, which cover the four other organs like leaves, reside in the first and uppermost location; thus, the pulse that indicates their path is necessarily light. Therefore, whoever wants to take a pulse at the aforementioned location will find it no more than three beans heavy, and it is detected on the surface of the skin and the surface of the hairs which grow on the skin. Thus, the lungs hold mastery over the skin and hair. The pulse is called *feu*, which means to swim.[194] The heart is below the lungs in the second position, and it holds mastery over the blood and veins. Thus, the pulses that indicate the path of the heart must be a little bit heavier. The fingers that take those pulses find that they are six beans heavy, and overflowing pulses are perceptible by pressing the veins. And so on with the rest, according to what has already been said.

Note, moreover, that the Chinese, when they attribute the name and nature of metals to the lungs, wanted to indicate the following things: that the lungs and the large intestines connected to them have those qualities that most especially agree with them, and which Metals themselves abound in above the others. Just as there are thickness, opacity, and coldness (for it is said that they use these <attributes> to produce water, which is especially cold), so too, as regards that quality through which metals resound and are vocal, these are things that most especially correspond to air. Thus, because air is extremely light, so too are the lungs are (which are closely connected to that quality), and their paths have lightness—that is, minimal or no heaviness. And so they say about the rest of the elementary qualities in the organs to which the nature of elements is attributed. In any event, let it suffice here to suggest that no one understands the genius of Chinese Doctors without understanding their reasoning on the things that they say.

---

[194] *natare*, literally, "to swim" "to float"

## CHAPTER TWELVE

*It is explained by what length of time the pulses (found in both right- and left-hand locations) and their circuits must be measured; and how, in taking pulses, anyone can make a determination on the good or bad health of the body and intestines by observing the aforementioned measure.*

After one has found the pulse locations and the circular motion of blood and spirits (from which pulses arise), there remains the measure of time, which, Galen says frankly, he could not find in the pulses. Not only have the Chinese have discovered those things that we related above (clearly unknown to European Physicians), but they even prescribed the measure of time (the noblest discovery in the Art) for pulses. Using this, they determine that one's health is good if the pulse regularly matches that measure, but if it falls short of that <measure> or exceeds it,[195] it means bad health.

Text: Every living person breathes, and in breathing, they exhale, or expel hot breath, bring in cold. Because pulses move at the time of exhalation and travel in the veins up to three finger-joints[196] in the human body; so too, at the time of breathing in, other <pulses have recourse> to three finger-joints.

This is because breathing in and breathing out constitute a single "breathing," and in the space of that time, the movement of pulses advances to six finger-joints in the human body.

And so, because a healthy man will produce day and night thirteen-thousand five-hundred[197] breaths, it follows that the motion of the pulses in the veins occupies a twenty-four hour

---

[195] *aut deficit, aut illam excedit*

[196] *decurrunt in venis ad tres articulos digitales*, exact sense unclear.

[197] *Spirationes...tredecim mille & quingentae*, not the normal way of saying 13,500 (should be *spirationum...tredecim milia & quingentae*). This could be 1,513 (literally, "thirteen one thousand and five hundred), but that seems unlikely; probably a problem in translating the Chinese into Latin. This repeats throughout the text, and I follow my standard of translation here.

period, according to both a man-made water-clock (such as the Chinese used), or rather, one-hundred quadrants.[198] This corresponds to a conversion of fifty homes (that is, celestial degrees) or Chinese constellations, by their assessment. But because radical wetness, being carried by its own motion in the middle of its circuit in the blood, advances during the time when the conversion of the heavens takes twenty-five homes; so too will primordial heat, carried in another half-circuit in the human body (or rather, in the veins), flow back and return in the spirits over the remaining time (when the conversion of the heavens takes place of the remaining twenty-five homes). Thus, both aforementioned things, in their turning and return, in their movement forward and back, use up and fill out the time of the whole conversion of the heavens, over fifty homes. At the same time, they arrive at the juncture of spirits and veins, the location where the paths of the six organs and of the six intestines (that is, the fonts of life) end and begin, as well as their motions and pulses, so that a rule is sought, not without reason, for taking pulses in the location in the hand where the aforementioned juncture exists.

Commentary: During exhalation (which is called *hŭ*), heat of a fiery nature is expelled; and then, during the subsequent inhalation, wet coldness of an airy nature is drawn in, or taken in, and it is called *hiĕ*; and that entails the entire act of breathing.[199] During a single breath, the pulses in the veins complete a journey in the body that extends six finger-joints. But just like the circulation of breaths, which encompasses 13,500 breaths, both day and night, during a 24-hour period; if the pulses in the human body advance six joints at each breath, the entire circuit of the pulses that move in the body will cover a span of 810 *chaṁ*. A *chaṁ* measure contains ten cubits; a cubit contains ten finger-joints; and a finger-joint also contains ten

---

[198] This seems to be another measure of time. According to my dictionary, a *quadrans* is a quarter of a day (six hours), but I suspect here it means a quarter of an hour (100 quarter-hours equals up to 25 hours, which is close to the other number given here).

[199] *ita integra existit spiratio*, "thus the whole of breathing exists."

parts. Again, because each path covers thirty-three *cham* measures and five *cuñ*, or finger-measures, and because over this entire extent of the paths the actual motion corresponds to a course of two heavenly homes and eight minutes (for the Chinese divide the heavens into fifty homes, which they also call degrees in their own fashion); then they also correspond to four quadrants and ten minutes according to a man-made water-clock, and thus the motion of fifty homes, and the whole time of twenty-four hours encompasses the entire circuit of the pulses as they course back and forth through the veins, at 810 measures. Thus, primordial heat (which is carried in the spirits inside and outside the blood in the veins[200]) takes that time which is given to the motion of 25 celestial homes, which is also twelve European hours. Likewise, radical wetness takes an equal course of another 25 homes and twelve European hours; so it happens that, once the fiftieth revolution of the celestial homes is complete, and a time of twenty-four hours has passed, the circuit of the pulses also is completed in the measure of the aforementioned distance. To make it clearer, note first: night and day (that is, the whole conversion of the heavens over fifty homes, which corresponds to twelve Chinese hours and twenty-four European hours) is measured by breathing-times, the whole course of which in a healthy man contains 13,500 breaths. Then, in your average healthy person, there happens to be found in the veins four or five pulses, over the course of one breath.[201] Thus it follows that there are no fewer than 54,000 vein-pulses over the day and night (or within 24 hours); or no more than 67,500. Because the motion of the heavens and the time and pulses' circulation match up to one another and are equal, it follows that, when a circular motion has a pulse that is neither slower nor faster than the motion of the heavens itself—that is, it should have neither more nor fewer pulses than we have indicated already; then everything is also right in the body. But if the circulation of pulses drops or increases—that is, if there are that many fewer slow pulses because of their slowness, or that many

---

[200] Exact meaning unclear.
[201] *intervallo*, literally, "during the interval (of)..." I translate it as "over the course (of)."

more because of their swiftness, they may perceive that a man is sick, and his organs and intestines and their paths are in disharmony because of this disagreement between the pulses and the motion of the heavens; for the Chinese believe that the circular motion of human life is the closest to celestial <motion>, which they believe to be the most regular and perfect of all things; and so, the standard model for all other motions. And so, because both radical wetness and primordial heat advance at each breath up to six finger-joints in the blood and spirits, movement is accomplished over the course and during the time of 13,500 breaths; and so it is necessary for the circulation of blood and spirits in the human body to comprise 810 *chaṁ* measures. The circular beginning of primordial heat in the blood (from the path of the lungs) comes from the Chinese hour (which is the third and fourth hour after midnight, when they believe that man was first formed in the nature of things out of muddy earth, just as woman was at the third and fourth hours of the evening) up until the sixth hour of the afternoon (which is the first and second hours, inclusively). Thus, the beginning of radical wetness comes from the third and fourth hours of the afternoon, up until the first and second hours after midnight, inclusively; because <it is> a complete circuit of two motions or pulses of radical wetness and primordial heat, which pulses begin in the right-hand location (called the mouth and spring of spirits) and end in the same place, so that they again begin at the third and fourth Chinese hours of the morning. Thus, Chinese doctors teach that the pulse travels from this right-hand location at the same time, and that one must use that to make determinations on the proper or deficient condition of the human body. This reveals with certainty, they say, at the designated location and time, the motions and conditions of the twelve paths of radical wetness and primordial heat; for spirits of radical wetness (meaning vital spirits) have not yet been dispersed; and the spirits of primordial heat (meaning animal spirits) have not yet been so disturbed, because they first begin to move from that place and at that time. Likewise, at the given time, food is not yet consumed, so the twelve paths are not refilled, and blood and spirits still remain in their natural location (not yet being disturbed), which happens at no other time. Therefore, just as *yñ* and *jam̄* (that is, heat and wetness) flow back and forth, according to the measure of the heavenly conversion, over fifty homes (or celestial degrees), so too do they do they flow back and forth over 24 hours and a distance of 810 *cham̄*; they found what things correspond to the cyclical[202] course of 13,500 breaths. Thus, based on a half-measure of the motion (25 celestial homes), and on a half measure of the time (twelve <European> hours, six Chinese), they believe that the measure of the space in which the circulation of veins exists, through the motion of *jâm* and *iñ* at half the distance, (which is 405 *cham̄* measures) and half the number of breaths, which totals 6,755.

One gathers from this that, during each of our hours (which correspond to half a Chinese hour), and for every two celestial homes (that is, one degree and five minutes), there are produced in a healthy man 562.5[203] breaths. But if the pulses are natural (because over every breath-span, there occur four or five pulses), no fewer than 2,250 pulses are found, or not much more than 2,812. In this interval, the blood and spirits (and in them, the *jâm* and *iñ*, heat and wetness)—that is, the life that results from them—advances three *cham̄* measures and seven *chĕ* (cubits) and five *cun* (finger-measures) through the aforementioned twisting span, through the winding paths in the human body. And so, because 140.5 breaths occur in a healthy man during a quarter-hour, it follows that there will be no fewer than 562 pulses, and no more than 702; and all the while, the blood and spirits in the human body will advance eight *cham* measures, four *chĕ*, and three *cun* (plus a little more).

A third thing: based on what we have discussed, just as the breaths in a healthy man correspond to the celestial circles in terms of time and consequently the motions of pulses in the veins correspond, so they are natural. But in a sick man, both

---

[202] *circulari*

[203] *spirationes...quingentae sexaginta duae & dimidia*, literally, "five hundred sixty two spirits and a half <part>." This construction repeats throughout.

breaths and pulse-motions always either fall short or surpass the typical number of breaths. Thus, just as the basis for recognizing something slanted is something straight, and the standard or basis for recognizing an unequal surplus or deficit is something equal, by the same rationale, a healthy man's regular or natural breaths and pulses, when properly observed, reveal the irregular and atypical breaths and pulses of sick men. Thus, the Chinese want the Doctor to be healthy, so that he can make determinations about others' illnesses according to what they say, lest a sick Doctor first attempt to cure himself. The reason for saying this, the Chinese will provide shortly. At the time of breathing for a healthy man, there are no fewer than four and no more than five breaths. But in a weak man, it is absolutely certain that there are fewer than four or more than five. From these pulses, they say that one can detect diseases, as well as the risk of death, and even death itself and its cause. Therefore, since a sick Doctor he lacks the breathing of a healthy man (which includes the measure of the heavens and of regular time, and the measure of a healthy man's breath), it is likely that regular pulses in a healthy person and irregular pulses in a sick person (whether in himself or another) should be normal,[204] and <the doctor> will easily think that it is another illness, unless by chance he is gifted, because of his great experience, in taking pulses of irregular measure, time, and breath-span; only thus would he be able to determine his own health, that of a sick man, and anyone else.

A fourth thing: the Chinese have found circulation not only in the blood and spirits, but in what comes out of them: pulses (which they measure by certain little breaks[205] in breathing). The circulation completely corresponds to a span of 24 hours, as well as to the complete conversion of the heavens; but the Chinese also found that is has a yearly circulation of blood and spirits; that is, over twelve lunar months, according to the seasons and changes of the year; that is, they distinguished the pulses of the twelve paths and the sources of the organs and intestines; and

---

[204] Grammar unclear.
[205] *morulas*, literally, "little delays," "little breaks"

not only did they declare that the long-lasting pulses share in the nature of the twelve paths and sources from which they arise (so that they can reveal their disposition), but they even assigned the pulses to some organs and the intestines and their paths according to the seasons of the year and the change that occurs then. In fact, they made note of the shortfalls, decreases, and growths of such pulses, as we shall show below.

Thus, just as the first long-lasting motion is called from east to west, and the second from west to east, so in a similar fashion one can connect the motion of the first moveable thing (over twenty-four hours) and the motion of its snatching,[206] so to speak.

It follows from what has been said that the extent of the veins in the human body is 800 *cham* measures. But in the designated pulse-location, according to the aforementioned circular motion, the measure of what was caused[207] is 13,500 breaths in a healthy. There is another measure for this measure: a circular revolution[208] of fifty celestial homes. But the artificial measure of this motion and time in a water clock contains a full one hundred fourths. There remains only to explain the measure of the pulses, one at a time.

---

[206] *raptus*, literally the act of taking, seizing, or snatching; "a snatching," "a taking"

[207] *causatorum*

[208] *circumvolution in orbem*, literally, "turning around into a sphere"

## CHAPTER THIRTEEN

*The circulation and motion of blood and spirits (or rather, the pulses, which complete their circular movement in a single day and night) through certain numbers of breaths, through a calculated movement of heavenly homes, and finally, through the measurement and example of hours and quadrants.*

W e have said that the circulation of blood and spirits ends where it begins and is completed in the right-hand *cun keu* location (where the pulse belongs to the lung-path) and its course finally begins in the morning of any given day, from which is becomes quite clear that, over the course of a day and night—24 hours—the pulses that begin from the movement of blood and spirits end at the same time and place. We shall now enumerate, one by one, the recorded measurements of this circular motion of blood and spirits (pulses), with the addition of the paths through which they travel, and the locations where they are found. Note first that the Chinese measure day and night (one full conversion of the heavens) in twelve hours, except when they use a water-clock of a hundred quadrants, which are no doubt smaller than ours. Therefore, by reducing both the water-clock and the twelve Chinese hours to the calculation of our time, the time taken by day and night will be twenty-four of our hours. Thus, one Chinese hour encompasses two of ours, and half a Chinese hour will be a whole one of ours—and according to the water-clock, four quadrants and ten minutes, at which time the heavenly spheres advance two homes (degrees) and eight minutes.

Having noted this carefully, pay attention to the following circulation demonstrated over its own hours in the follow example. That it may be easier to understand, I omit the example of saying things in a single Chinese hour.

At the third European hour after midnight—which in China corresponds to half an hour (called *im*) on a clock, and likewise to four quadrants and ten minutes on a water-clock, and to two Chinese homes (degrees) and five minutes in the conversion of the heavens—the lungs propagate[209] radical wetness to the hands through the spirits and blood. It is called the path of great radical wetness.

In the first point of the right hand, the *cun* pulses, which indicate the path and condition of the lungs (because, you see, at that aforementioned time, 562.5 breaths are completed in a healthy man, and the spirits and blood in the veins of the human body move 33 *châm* measures, seven *chĕ*, and five *cûn*) occur in a healthy man no fewer than 2250 times, and not much more than 2813 times.

At the fourth hour of the morning—which corresponds to another Chinese half-hour (*im*), and to four quadrants, ten minutes; or (if you wish to multiply by additions to what came before,[210] as we ourselves do with China in the example), it corresponds to eight quadrants and twenty minutes on the aforementioned clock, and to two Chinese degrees and five minutes, or rather, (by addition) four degrees and twenty minutes—the same lungs propagate radical wetness through the aforementioned hand-path. The regular pulses that reveal the path in the same right-hand location number 562.5 in a healthy man; or rather, (by addition) 1125, and the same spirits, along with the blood, move 33 *châm* and five *chĕ* in the veins. The regular pulses, I say, number no more than 5625, nor less than 4500; and so it is shown, by adding or multiplying the previous parts of each hour in the order shown in the model, that they agree with the latter ones.[211]

At the fifth hour, which corresponds to half a Chinese *mao*, twelve quadrants on a clock, and six degrees 24 minutes *cum* in the sky, in the large intestines, they propagate *jâm*, natural heat, through the blood and the spirits away from the hands. It is called the path of pure and bright heat. In the first point of the right hand, regular pulses indicate this path and the condition of the

---

[209] *propagant*, literally, "drive forward," I think the mechanic would now be called "pumping."

[210] *per additiones ad priora multiplicare*, the exact sense is unclear

[211] Meaning unclear.

large intestines (since there occur 1687 breaths at the given time; and spirits, along with blood of veins, move up to 101 *cham*, two *chĕ*, and five *cùn*). These pules then number no fewer than 6,750, and no more than 8437.

At the sixth hour, which corresponds to a full Chinese *Mao* and sixteen quadrants and a little more; and likewise to eight degrees in the heavens and 32 minutes, the same large intestines propagate primordial head through the aforementioned path from the hand to the head, and when one takes 2,250 breaths and the vein spirits, along with the blood, move 135 *cham*, then the regular pulses number no fewer than 9000 and no more than 11,250.

At the seventh hour, which corresponds to half a Chinese *Xin*, and to 22 quadrants, and to 10 degrees 40 minutes, the stomach propagates primordial heat to the feet. This is called the path to the feet of bright primordial heat. In the second point in the right hand, they propagate the condition of both the path and the organ (when 2813.5 breaths are complete, and the spirits, along with the blood, travel 168 *cham*, 7 *chĕ*, and 5 *cuñ*). Regular pulses number no fewer than 11250 and no more than 14062.

At the eighth hour, which corresponds to a full Chinese *Xin*, and to 26 quadrants, and to 12 degrees, 48 minutes, the same stomach propagates primordial heat to the same path in the feet. At this time, after 3375 breaths are complete, and the spirits, along with the blood, move 202 *chm*, 5 *chĕ* in the veins, regular pulses number no fewer than 13500 and no more than 16875.

At the ninth hour, which corresponds to half a Chinese *sú*, according to the clock, to 28 quadrants in the heavens, and to 14 degrees, 56 minutes, the spleen propagates radical wetness to the heart, and this is called the great path of radical wetness in the feet or from the feet. In the second point in the hand, they propagate the condition of this path and the stomach (when 3937.5 breaths have been taken, and the spirits along with the blood move 236 *cham*, 2 *chĕ*, 5 *cun* in the veins). There are regular pulses, which number no fewer than 15780 and no more than 19687.

At the tenth hour, which corresponds to a full Chinese *su*, or rather, 32 quadrants of the clock (plus a little), and to 16 degrees, 64 minutes, the same spleen propagates radical wetness through the aforementioned path in the feet, and when 4500 breaths have been taken, and the spirits along with the blood move 270 *cham̃*, the regular pulses indicate its condition, which number no fewer than 18000 and no more than 22500.

At the eleventh hour, which corresponds to half a Chinese *ú*, 34 quadrants of the clock, and to 18 degrees and 7 minutes in the heavens, the heart propagates radical wetness to the hands, and this is called the path of diminished radical wetness in the hands. It is situated in the first location *cun* in the left hand, when 6062.5 breaths have been taken, and when spirits and blood in the veins move 303 *cham*, 7 *chĕ*, 5 *cuñ*, the regular pulses give indication, which number no fewer than 20250, no more than 25300.

At the twelfth hour (noon), which corresponds to a complete Chinese *ú*, and to 40 quadrants of the clock, and to 20 degrees, 8 minutes in the heavens, the same heart propagates radical wetness to the hands. When 5625 breaths have been taken at that aforementioned time, and when spirits and blood move 337 *cham* and 5 *che* in the veins, there occur no fewer than 22500 pulses, no more than 28124.

At the first hour, which corresponds to half a Chinese *ui*, and to 44 quadrants of the clock, and to 22 degrees, 2 minutes in the heavens, the small intestines propagate heat to the hands, and this is called the path of great primordial heat in the hands.in the first point *cun* in the left hand, when 6187 breaths have been taken at the aforementioned time, and spirits along with blood move in the veins 371 *cham*, 2 *chĕ*, and 5 *cun*, there are no fewer than 24750 and no more than 30937 regular pulses, which indicate the constitution of a healthy man.

At the second hour, which corresponds to a complete Chinese *ui*, and to 46 quadrants of the clock, plus a little more; and to 24 degree 20 minutes in the heavens, the same small intestines propagate heat away from the hands, and at the time when 6750 breaths have been taken and the spirits in the body, along with the blood, move 405 *cham*, there are no fewer than 27000 regular pulses, and no more than 33750.

At the third hour, which corresponds to half a Chinese *Xin*, 52 quadrants, and to 26 degrees and 54 minutes, the ureters propagate natural heat to the feet; this is called the path of great heat for the feet. In the third point *chĕ* in the right hand, regular pulses indicate the condition of this path, when 7312 breaths have been taken, and spirits along with blood move 438 *cham*, 7 *chĕ*, 5 *cun*. These pulses number no fewer than 29250 and no more than 36562.

At the fourth hour, which corresponds to a full Chinese *Xin*, 56 quadrants, and to 29 degrees and 6 minutes in the heavens, the same ureters propagate heat to the feet; and when they have completed 7875.5 breaths, and the spirits along with blood move 472 *cham* and 5 *chĕ* , there are no fewer than 31500 regular pulses, and no more than 39375.

At the fifth hour, which corresponds to half a Chinese *yeû*, 60 quadrants of the clock, and to 31 degrees and 4 minutes in the heavens, the bladder (kidneys) propagate radical wetness from the feet; this is called the path of diminished radical wetness for the feet. A man's health is diagnosed in the third point *chĕ* in the left hand, at the time when they have completed 8437.5 breaths, and the spirits along with blood are propagated 506 *cham* and 2 *chĕ*, 5 *cùn* in the veins. There are no fewer than 33950 regular pulses, and no more than 421887.

At the sixth hour, which corresponds to a full Chinese *yeû*, 62 quadrants of the clock, and to 33 degrees and twelve minutes, the same bladder (kidneys) propagate radical wetness from the feet, which indicate the health of this path. When 9000 breaths have been taken, and the spirits along with blood have traveled

540 *cham* in the body, there are no fewer than 36000 regular pulses, and no more than 45000.

At the seventh hour, which corresponds to half a Chinese *Siō*, 66 quadrants of the clock, and to 35 degrees, 25 minutes in the heavens, the gate of life propagates radical wetness to hands; this is called the path of defective radical wetness for the hands. The condition of this path is indicated in the third point *chĕ* of the right hand. When 9572.5 breaths have been taken in a healthy man, and the spirits along with blood have moved 573 *cham*, 7 *che*, and 5 *cún* in the veins, there are no fewer than 38250 regular pulses, and no more than 47812.

At the eighth hour, which corresponds to a full Chinese *Sio*, to 70 quadrants plus some, and to 37 degrees and 28 minutes, the same gate of life propagates radical wetness to the hands, when 10125 breaths have been taken, and spirits along with blood move 607 *cham* and 5 *che* in the veins. There are no fewer than 40500 regular pulses, and no more than 50625.

At the ninth hour, which corresponds to half a Chinese *hai*, to 72 quadrants, and to 39 degrees and 36 minutes, the third part of the body propagates heat away from the hands. This is called the path of diminished heat for the hands. The condition of this path is declared in the third point of the right hand, *chĕ*, when 10607.5 breaths have been taken, and spirits along with blood move 641 *cham*, 2 *chĕ*, and 5 *cùn*. There are no fewer than 42750 regular pulses, and no more than 53437.

At the tenth hour, which corresponds to a full Chinese *hai*, and to 74 quadrants, and to 40 degrees and 44 minutes, the same third part of the body propagates heat away from the hands, and when 11250 breaths have been taken in a healthy man, and spirits along with blood travel 675 *cham* in the veins, there are no fewer than 45000 regular pulses, and no more than 56250.

At the eleventh hour, which corresponds to half a Chinese *Cù*, 80 quadrants, and to 43 degrees and 52 minutes, the gall bladder propagates natural heat to the feet. This is called the path of diminished heat for the feet. In the second point *quan*, in the left hand, the condition of this path is indicated, when 11813 breaths have been taken, and when the spirits in the veins have travelled 78 *cham*, 7 *chě*, 5 *cùn*. There are no fewer than 47280 regular pulses, and no more than 59062.

At the twelfth hour, which corresponds to complete Chinese *cù*, 90 quadrants, and to 45 degrees and 6 minutes in the heavens, the same gall bladder propagates heat to the feet, and when 12375 breaths have been taken, and the spirits along with the blood in the veins have advances 742 *cham*, 5 *chě*, there are no fewer than 49500 regular pulses, and no more than 61875.

At the first hour, which corresponds to half a Chinese *cheŭ*, and to 96 quadrants of the clock, and to 98 degrees, the liver propagates radical wetness from the feet. This is called the path of defective radical wetness for the feet. In the second point *quan* of the left hand, the condition of this path is indicated, at the aforementioned time when 12937.5 breaths have been taken and the spirits along with blood have travelled 776 *cham*, 2 *chě*, and 5 *cun*. There are no fewer than 51750 regular pulses, and no more than 64687.

At the second hour after midnight, which corresponds to a full Chinese *cheu*, and to 100 quadrants of the clock, and to 50 degrees in the heavens, the same liver propagates radical wetness away from the feet, and at the aforementioned time, when 13500 breaths have been taken, and spirits along with the blood have moved in the veins 810 *cham*, there are no fewer than 54000 pulses, and no more than 67500. And so on in a circle, with things revolving according to the revolution of the heavens and the duration of breaths (by clock) and motions in space; so too does the regularity of the veins and pulses also revolve in a healthy person,[212] from which health can be determined at night and in the day; indeed, at individual hours, and not only in the entire body, but even in individual organs and intestines.

---

[212] Exact meaning unclear, but it seems to be drawing a parallel between the heavenly cycle and the circulatory system.

Note carefully that, according to the double motion of the heavens—that is, the daily motion, which is 24 hours, and the yearly motion—not only are daily pulses found, but yearly ones, and they differ according to the difference between the four seasons in man, and they are caused by blood and spirits. For this reason, Chinese doctors teach that, each organ and intestine—or rather, for each pulse location—possesses within it also its own particular variations, according to its time and the season of the year. Thus, in spring, pulses are different than in the summer, and in winter; different than in autumn. So it happens that, according to the varying nature of the pulses, the names given to the pulses also vary. They want the measures— both of the heavens and of the clock, both of breaths and of the length of the pulse[213]—at whatever time of the year they occur, to be completely the same natural measures. But if they see that the pulses of one season (either past or future) creep in place of a connatural pulse, they realize that a person is sick because of that. And just as they recognize that a person is faring poorly if their daytime pulses surpass or fall short of the determined measure of time and of the number of breaths in a healthy person, or of the disordered nature of the pulses; so too would they determine that a person's life is also being affected negatively if they found the circulation, if they found disturbances or changes in the annual and monthly increases and decreases in the spring, summer, autumnal, and winter season.

But, in order for anyone to easily ascertain the measure of pulses and from it to identify health and illnesses, let us move on to the next chapter.

---

[213] *spatii pulsuum*

## CHAPTER FOURTEEN

*How one can determine the measure of regular pulses in an easy manner, and how, from that measure, health, illnesses, and death itself can be identified with no trouble.*

This chapter is foremost of wonderful use and utility, as too are those that follow—of course, whoever takes even modest note of what we shall say will be able to pass judgment on life and health, on diseases and their causes, on death (even which shall come), and that with almost no trouble. Let us reveal the secret.

We have said that the period of 13,500 breaths completes the course of measures that the blood and spirits create, for during that time, the pulses are measured that were caused by the circulatory motion that was mentioned. But because it is exceedingly difficult to take pulses through an entire day and night, even after a great delay of breaths—not to mention taking it at the hour, or even at the quadrant—[214]and it would be a most tedious task to take pulses which happen over the course of so many breaths during that time. It has proven beneficial to prescribe a rather short interval in which the regular pulses can be determined, both failing and surpassing.

Next, Chinese Doctors argue that whoever is going to take another's pulse should be completely healthy himself, free from troubles and cares, as well as any other serious weakness; for it could happen that they could have a connatural breath. Here, the Doctor uses an interval of one, two, three, and up to nine breaths, because he himself finds in the pause between breaths[215] no more than 5 pulses, but no fewer than four, when he takes pulses in locations in each hand, he will definitely say that they are the regular pulses for that person, and that he is healthy. The reasoning for this is extremely subtle, as follows: Breath, they say, consists of exhalation (that is, the ejection of air) and inhalation (that is, the drawing in of air). Therefore, if you count

---

[214] Grammar a little unclear, this seems to be the sense.
[215] *mora spirationum*, literally, "the pause of breathings."

two pulses in the same of a breath (note that this will indicate the condition of the paths of the heart and lungs); and then, in the span of drawing in breath, you again find two pulses, it is understood that they are the pulses of the paths of the bladder (kidneys) and liver. Because these paths intersect one another and accomplish a certain harmony of life between each other, they indicate the same <path> through the aforementioned pulses, in the given number (no less), up to the aforementioned interval which is found in a healthy person. And if it should happen, in the space of one breath, that there are five pulses, one should understand that the fifth pulse indicates the path of the stomach, and is in the middle of the pulses, just as the stomach is also in the middle of the organs. But the pulses at the interval of a full breath are said to indicate a person's good health, such that they reveal the internal condition of five organs (the heart, lungs, stomach, bladder, and liver) by the number of five beats[216] (and so on with each pulse location; but such that the beginning of the beats—or rather, their number—is attributed to that organ and path at whose location pulses are taken). And so on in order.

Next, because we have said that a person is shown to be healthy by four pulses over the course of a single breath, you must understand that it happens thus because those four beats not only indicate the status of the four organs (the heart, lungs, bladder, and liver), but even of the stomach (whose spirits are the foundation of all pulses). Thus, those same four pulses reveal the properties that it has hidden within itself. Therefore, if you find either four or five pulses in the course of one breath, you will pronounce the person healthy. But if you note the pulses decreasing—that is, there are fewer pulses over the count of a whole breath, you will no doubt declare the body badly afflicted. The reason is at hand, because the regular number of pulses (that were just designated) damages or even destroys the concord of life, whether by its excess or its deficiency.

*But let us hear the Chinese text:*

---

[216] *ictus*, literally, "strokes," "welts," "lashes," here meaning pulse-beats.

Why are some pulses called more, or surpassing, but others are called fewer or deficient[217]? Because, of course, if over the course of exhalation or inhalation, there are only two pulses, they will indicate that the person is healthy—that is, that they are faring well. But if there are three pulses over the same span, they are said to be *li kim*, wandering off the path. If there are four pulses, they are said to be taking away its perfection and integrity, and if there are five pulses over that same time, they are said to be dangerous and mortal. If six, they are said to be severing life. These are all the surpassing pulses.

Why are they called few or deficient pulses? Because if, during a single breath (out or in), there is only a single pulse, it is the same thing, and is said to be wandering from the path. But if, in the span of two breaths, one whole pulse occurs, it is said to be carrying away the integrity of life. And if one whole pulse happens during the course of three breaths, it is called mortal. Finally, if a single pulse occurs over the course of four breaths, it is said to be severing life. And these are called the deficient pulses. Then the pulses, which are more or surpassing, begin from the lower quarter up to the highest; and the pulses which are few or descending run from the upper to the lower.

Commentary: As is said in the text, if there are two pulses over the course of breathing out, they indicate that a person is healthy—if, obviously, in the course of one whole breath there are at least four pulses (for breathing consists of exhalation and inhalation). And so, when he counts the number of pulses from one part of breathing (that is, inhalation), he wants it to be the same from the other part (exhalation). And so it is for the remaining pulses, whether surpassing or deficient. But what is said about deficient pulses, if one pulse happens over the course of inhalation, it should mean that, if you count only two pulses in the time it takes for a whole breath, such pulses are called *pai me*; that is, destroying and corrupting. These two pulses from among the deficient ones, and those six pulses from among the

---

[217] *deficientes*

surpassing ones, when they occur[218] over the course of one whole breath, are called *li him*, wandering away from the ordinary and natural path, from which they determine that people are sick.

If there are seven or eight surpassing or more pulses during the course of one whole breath, and only a single one occurs from among the deficient or fewer pulses over the course of one entire breath, both of them are said to be *to cuom*, carrying away the integrity of life; because, of course, the spirits dominate and dry out the blood, and the bloom and vitality of life languishes, and its heat is violently taken away.

If, then, in the course of a single breath, you notice ten surpassing pulses, and if you notice only a single one of the deficient pulses over the course of one whole breath and a half (that is, of breathing out), it indicates that a person is ready for the grave,[219] for two such pulses are said to be mortal. But if, out of the surpassing pulses, you detect twelve over the course of one breath, know that the spirit is severed and separated. And if, out of the deficient pulses, only one occurs in the course of two whole breaths (and this pulse is said to be monstrous, and it indicates that life is separating—that is, the disposition of the organs is destroyed, and that by a deficient spirit), the soul departs, and death follows. These are the four pulses of death.

Text: Why do the sick have few or deficient pulses? Because, deficient pulses of the first sort (meaning when two pulses occur over the course of a whole breath; and they are called destroying pulses) damage the skin and make the hair fall off. Deficient pulses of the second sort (meaning when a single pulse occurs over the span of one breath; and this is called the pulse that takes away the integrity of life) damage the blood, and because it is emptied out and keeps very little of itself, it cannot animate and replenish[220] the organs and intestines. Deficient pulses of the third type (meaning when a single pulse happens over the course

---

[218] Not provided by the Latin, but I believe it is implied.

[219] *sepulchro subjici,* "to be subject to the grave."

[220] *irrigare,* literally, "irrigate"

of one whole breath and a half; and this is called the "mortal" pulse) damages and dries out the flesh; so it comes to pass that food and drink cannot fix a person's wasting. Deficient pulses of the fourth sort (meaning when a single pulse is detected in the span of two whole pulses; and this is called the monstrous pulse) damages the sinews—meaning, of course, their weakness or idleness cannot then be fixed. Deficient pulses of the fifth sort (meaning if a single pulse occurs over the span of two and a half breaths) damages the bones and dries out the marrow, so it comes to pass that a sick person is bound to bed and cannot again get up.

A similar fashion must be taken as concerns surpassing pulses, which by themselves also indicate diseases, but in determining the latter, they make the former go from the lower sections to the upper; that is, from those pulses that indicate dry bones and are the reason why a sick man cannot get up from bed until it comes to the wasting of the skin and hair-loss, for in deficient pulses, diseases climb in a certain way from the upper to the lower parts; that is, from the wasting of the skin to the loss of hair, up to the drying of the bones. Whatever pulse has either the one or the other[221] <pulses> that indicate the aforementioned progress of the diseases, you should believe that your death is looming presently.

Commentary: Of all the organs in the location of the upper region, the lungs have pride of place, as they cover the other organs with something like wings, and they take within the motions of all the paths. So it comes to pass that the path of the lungs is like the sea, with all the pulses ebbing and flowing,[222] to which it grants animate life and vital spirits and wherever it pours itself out, it grants superabundant enlivenment to the skin and hair.

Because diseases are indicated by deficient pulses, as one climbs in diseases from the upper to the lower regions, so too will the

---

[221] *hos vel illos*, meaning "deficient or surpassing pulses"
[222] *congregantis & reciprocantis omnes pulsus*, literally, "gathering together and turning back all pulses."

lungs (holding the chief-most position of all, and invigorating the skin and hair by its own path), because they have deficient pulses of the first sort. In the first location of the right hand, it is necessary for the skin to languish, and hair to fall out, from which disease and the bad health of the lungs is determined; as one descends to the inner parts, because the heart (which is the Lord of the blood) is below the lungs (which thus indicate defective pulses of the second sort), they thus indicate that the heart is faring poorly; that the blood is diminished, dried out, emptied; so follows wasting in the five organs and six intestines. And because the stomach also rests below the heart and takes in five spirits of sustenance (meaning: wheat, rice, beans), through which it gives extra nourishment to the flesh, within the organs and intestines; so do deficient pulses of the third sort indicate the injury with which the stomach is mightily afflicted, and it even appears from that that neither food nor drink are digested; necessarily, then, the flesh must languish and waste.

Again, because the liver (which is the workshop of blood) is roughly beneath the stomach, and maintains that blood, and attends to the heart, and likewise replenishes the nerves, and invigorates the nails. Deficient pulses of the fourth type indicate damage that the liver endures, which can be seen in the nerves, which, being remiss and loose, affect the whole body in a similar way.

Finally, because the bladder is lower than any of the other organs and maintains the paths of the five organs and six intestines by its spirits, it comes to pass that even the hairs themselves are invigorated by its path; the bones and marrow, too; and thus, deficient pulses of the fifth sort reveal injury and damage to the bladder, which the bones themselves indicate by being dried and withered. Accordingly, weakness in the body arises in the sick man, and a sluggishness of sleep; and he cannot again get himself up from bed.

These five sorts of deficient pulses indicate five types of diseases, and they do that by descending from the diseases of the upper organs to the diseases of the lower ones—meaning, from the lungs up to the bladder or kidneys. But the opposite happens with types of surpassing pulses, for the illnesses of lower organs climbs towards the illnesses of the upper organs (meaning, away from damage to the bladder towards damage to the lungs, as above).

Text: How shall we best treat the five types of deficient pulses already described? Quite well, in the following way: if you see that deficient pulses of the first sort indicate a disease of the lungs, you will restore the spirits of the lungs; if of the second sort, they indicate a disease of the heart, and you will adjust the motion of the spirits and blood. If they are of the third sort (indicating a disease of the stomach), the treatment will lie in the regulation of food and drink, by mixing hot and cold together. If they are of the fourth sort, showing a disease in the liver, you will need to induce a remission of the spirits.[223] If of the fifth sort, indicating a disease of the bladder, you should increase the qualities of the bladder that are used to identify it in the first place. At this is the method for providing treatment using the aforementioned pulses.

Commentary: Cold and cold food damage the lungs; thus, you should treat a disease of the lungs by restoring the spirits over which they hold power, for all pulses are detected through spirits and are reduced to a natural state; it is also from here that strength returns to the skin and hair. Lastly, sadness, anxiety, excessive thinking damages the heart, which holds power over the blood; thus, you should treat a disease of the heart by reducing the harmonic motion of blood and spirits. So it will happen that the veins are filled again with spirits and blood and go on to extend the natural motion of pulses.

Excessive food and drink, as well as great weariness, harm the spleen and stomach, for its qualities appear more every three months, according to the four seasons of the year. For this reason, one must treat this disease of the stomach with the tastes of food and drink, in agreement with the cold or war spirits of

---

[223] Exact meaning unclear.

the four seasons of the year, so that a reduction to its proper mixture can feed the flesh.

Excessive anger and choler[224] do excessive damage to the liver; in that case, you will treat the diseases of the liver if you eat sweet food: for instance, rice, which serves to create wine and is itself sweet; likewise <*bubula*>[225] and the fruit called *cao cu*, which is like prunes and other such fruits. This is because the liver has a swift, intense, and ardent nature and qualities. But tastes—especially sweetness—since they are of an earthy character, have remiss virtues, and so they ease the liver's effort, bringing it about that the nerves (over which the liver hold power) are moderated. A delay or pause during the day in wet places, as well as a violent struggle of forces, harm the bladder or kidneys; but the bladder is the foundation of bodily nourishment. You will be able to treat those illnesses with table salt; for thus you will restore its nature and the spirits by which it nourishes the bones and the marrow of the bones.

That is the rule for treating the five sorts the five sorts of deficient pulses; and it follows from here how one must proceed with those diseases that indicate the five types of surpassing pulses.

Text: Certain pulses have three beats during a single exhalation, and the same number during a single inhalation. Likewise, some have four beats during one exhalation, and four too during one inhalation; five and five, six and six—some pulses have one beat during one exhalation, and one beat during one inhalation; likewise, one beat over two exhalations and one beat over two inhalations; likewise, one single beat over two exhalations and two inhalations.

But how will you recognize them and determine diseases from them? I answer: if the two pulse-beats occur over the course of exhalation, and another two over the course of inhalation (these

---

[224] *cholera*

[225] Not sure what this refers to; it seems like it should be a food, which might make it a transliteration of the Greek βουβάλιον, "wild cucumber."

being generally neither large nor small), you shall call them equal pulses. And if you detect three beats over the course of exhalation, and another three beats over the course of inhalation, a disease is already beginning; because if the earlier pulse-beats are great, and the latter ones small, you should know that the head is suffering, and that the eyes are heavy and darkened. If, however, the earlier pulse-beats are small and the latter ones great, you should know that the chest is filled up; and that the spirits, or rather, respiration, is tight.

Commentary: If over the course of a single whole breath (which consists of exhalation and inhalation) there are four pulse-beats, and they are neither terrible great nor terrible small, but are modest, they indicate that a person is healthy. But if you notice six beats over this time, the pulse is fast, and it suggests the beginning of disease.

If the first pulse-beats (meaning in the first location) are great, and the latter pulses (meaning in the third location) are small (because the first pulse-location is like heaven and governs the topmost part, from the chest to the head), it shows pain in the brain,[226] and in the eyes, when they move, heaviness and darkness. But if the first pulses or beats are small and the latter large—that is, after the first pulse-location; if in the second location, which points towards the middle or second region in the body (which is called "man"), they show that the chest is filled and the knees are heavy, and thus that sluggishness dwells in the feet.

Text: Four beats over the course of one exhalation and four other beats during inhalation indicate a great illness. If the pulses are superabundant and great, the sick complain about the irritation and restlessness; but if they are deep and subtle, there is pain within the belly; and if they are fast and sharp,[227] they indicate damage from the cold; but if, at last, the pulses detected are dull

---

[226] *capitis in cerebro dolorem*, literally, "pain of the head in the brain."

[227] *Crebro-acuti*, a created compound adjective, I believe, from *creber*, "crowded," and *acutus*, "sharp," "keen."

and thin,[228] one must determine that there are many cold humors within.

Commentary: Eight beats over the course of one breath indicate that injury has taken hold, and because they are superabundant and great, the disease is in the path of threefold primordial heat, because many pulses are made because of great heat, and they indicate that the heart and chest are filled with sadness and annoyance and restlessness because of the cold and heat that has arisen. But if the pulses are deep and subtle, the illness comes from the path of threefold radical wetness, for much wetness, holding power over the cold, causes and brings about pain in the bones, so that spirits of primordial heat are harmed by excessive external heat. Finally, if the pulses are dull and infrequent, they indicate that there is too little blood, and that there is an abundance of vapors, since there is too much cold; and thus a growl is made within the guts.

Text: Five beats being detected over the course of exhalation and another five over the course of inhalation indicate that a sick person is seriously afflicted. So, if they are deep and subtle and come by night, and then go away shaky and great,[229] but appear neither great nor small by day, although the disease be extremely difficult, it can be cured. But so long as they are only small and great, you will cure them with great difficulty, for those great, subtle pulses by day are numerous.

Commentary: A pulse of eight beats is called <the pulse> of separation; nine beats, mortal. Those words are suggestive.[230] But if there are pulses of ten beats over the course of a full breath, the sick person is ready for the grave, for the illness is most difficult and most troublesome. If the pulses are deep and subtle, wetness is dramatically increased; if they are abundant and great, heat is dramatically increased by day. If they are

---

[228] *Obtuso-rari*, same as above.

[229] *nutantes & magni*; *nutantes* literally means "nodding." Maybe a typo for *natantes*, "floating"?

[230] *Ista verba innuunt*, literally, "those words nod forward." *Innuere* comes to mean "suggest" or "intimate," but the exact sense is unclear.

neither great, nor small, nor abundant, nor deep, the illness, though it be difficult and fierce, can be cured. But if the pulses are inconstant—that is, they are sometimes great, sometimes small; sometimes fast, sometimes slow—it is a sign that certain death is looming.

Text: Six beats being detected over the course of one exhalation, and the same number over the course of one inhalation, indicate death. If those pulse-beats are deep, death occurs at night; if they are abundant and great, they show that the sick person will die by day.

Commentary: Twelve beats over the course of one breath show that the spirit or life is destroyed. The reason for this is: because primordial heat is in far too great supply.[231] If the pulses are determined to be deep and subtle, and night is looming, it follows that the sick person will die on that very night. But if they are great and abundant, the person will die by day, for that is when radical wetness separates from primordial heat. Let what has been said suffice for the many pulses (the surpassing ones), for what follows concerns the few, or deficient pulses.

Text: One beat over the course of exhalation, and another beat during inhalation, is characteristic of a deficient pulse. Whoever has this, although he may be able to walk, he cannot get out— no, he will collapse into his bed in the end, because the blood and spirits are not adequate.

Commentary: One type of deficient pulses that has only two beats over the course of one whole breath, and another type that has only a single beat over the course of one breath, is said to be characteristic of corrupt pulses, because the organs and intestines suffer damage from exhaustion and lose their perfection, vigor, and nourishment, and that because the blood and spirits are inadequate.

Text: One beat over the course of two exhalations, and another single beat over the course of another two inhalations, are said

---

[231] *omnino nimius*, literally, "altogether excessive."

to be without soul,[232] because such a person is definitely going to die. Although a sick person may be able to get around, he takes the name of "living corpse."

Commentary: When a single pulse occurs over the course of a full breath, the soul looks to primordial heat and the body to radical wetness, and when heat too is failing, the soul departs; and the sick man, although he moves and gets around, is called a living corpse.

Text: If the first pulse-location in the hands has a pulse, and if the third pulse-location is lacking one, that man must vomit; if he does not vomit, he certainly will die. But if the upper location is lacking a pulse and one is found in the third location, although the difficulty and pain of the ailment will be very great, it shows that no lethal damage will accrue, because a person that regularly has a pulse in the third place is like a tree that has its roots, branches, and leaves—if the branches and leaves dry up, the roots still remain, from which all the rest are fueled. Therefore, one must not lose hope.

Commentary: If the third location is lacking a pulse, it is a sign that the upper regions are toiling with the defect of being overstuffed. Thus, it is necessary either to relieve that fullness by vomiting, or for the innermost parts to be suffocated by the spirits that arise there; then comes death. The pulse in the third location of the left hand aims at the path of the bladder; that in the third location of the right hand aims at the path of the gate of life, for both conceal spirits, because those are their location and source. Therefore, if the first location in the hands lacks any pulse, and one appears in the third location, it is clear that the original spirits endure and are maintained. Thus, it readily follows that whoever has those pulses is not yet dying.

First, it follows: Why are deficient pulses of the first sort (as when only a single pulse occurs over the course of a whole breath) and surpassing pulses (as when six pulses occur over the

---

[232] *sine anima*, literally, "without breeze," but *anima* usually refers to breath (as the breath of life) or the soul (by the same principle).

course of a breath) said to be "deviating from the normal path"? Because, if it happens over the course of a whole breath that the spirits and blood in the human body move up to six finger-measures, the surpassing pulses would over that same span complete seven measures. So it follows that they complete their circuit more and more quickly, so that something like a third part of the normal time remains (because of the speed of the pulses).

On the one hand, in deficient pulses, it is necessary for them to be slowed by the same amount and to fall short of the regular time; so it is clear that both deviate from the ordinary path. In a like fashion must one discuss both deficient and surpassing pulses of the second, third, fourth, and fifth type. By running through them, you will find that everyone you see to be deficient will be so from the measures of breaths in a healthy man; likewise, in the heavenly revolution, and likewise in the determined time of a water-clock, and that over an equal course and span of veins in the human body (as we indicated above). On the other hand, you will find that they surpass those measures in surpassing pulses.

Now a single thing must be considered as we move along: whether the prescribed pulses of the aforementioned measures are found in people of every age and sex—whether the same pulse measure exists in child and adult, fat and thin, tall and short, slow and swift, male and female—or, at any rate, whether the quality of those pulses is varied in them, and whether at some point the pulses stop and change, and what the cessation or change means; finally, whether a pulse that is constant at a certain number can provide certain information on times, death, or disease?

## CHAPTER FIFTEEN

*Whether the measure of breaths as related is the same in children and adults; whether the quality of pulses is the same in man and women, thin and fat, tall and little, slow and swift; and whether the pulses stop, and what knowledge of the time, diseases, and death someone can come to from that rest, at a certain number of pulses?*

Text: In boys aged three to five years, over the course of a whole exhalation and inhalation, one must note the pulse carefully; for if there are eight beats over the aforementioned time, they are well; if nine, they have an internal malady; if ten or twelve, the disease is difficult, but exceedingly so; if there are sometimes short beats, sometimes long, sometimes small, or great, they are not without a risk of death, and they show that the ailment is deep-rooted.

Commentary: The pulses of children[233] are entirely different from those of adults. Likewise, if a tall person has a subtle pulse, and a thin and slender person has a great one; a joyous person has a full pulse, and a sad person an empty pulse; an excited person has a remiss pulse, and a heavy and slow person has a quick pulse; a rustic and thick man has a delicate pulse, a delicate man, a thick pulse; a short person, and of small stature, has a long pulse, while a skinny person has a great pulse, surpassing their long body; and a hardy person has a thin pulse; a fat person a small pulse; or sick person, suffering from diarrhea, has as well a great pulse of blood. Almost all these pulses are signs of Death, or they indicate a most dangerous illness. For that reason, a person who intends to take pulses should take careful note of whether a person is tall, short, swift, slow, and so on, and whether or not the pulses correspond in three pulse locations in each hand, each one's inherent state or disposition.

Now, could there be a question of whether the pulses in a man and woman observe the same location and measures? The

---

[233] *Parvulorum*, literally, "little tiny persons," but I think the distinction here is between small children and full-grown adults.

Michal Boym

Chinese Doctors answer that, for men, the third location in each hand, called *che*, always has weaker pulses; for women though, the first location *cun* in either hand has weaker pulses, and the third location stronger pulses. Therefore (they say), if you find in a man that the third location *che* has firm pulses, you should know that that man has a woman's pulse; and this pulse in a man comes from deficient <pulses>. But if you find a weak pulse in the third location *che* in a woman, know that the woman has a man's pulse, and these pulses come from surpassing <pulses>. Thus, you will determine that both man and woman are faring poorly.

Text: Some pulses are natural or ordinary, others are against nature and extraordinary. Why are men's and women's pulses opposite? Because, the first man began to live at the start of the hour *ym* (that is, the third and fourth hour after midnight), and this hour points to *yam*, primordial heat; and the first woman began to live at the hour of *Xin* (that is, the third and fourth hour after noon) which points towards radical wetness. Thus, a man's first or principal pulse is found under the second location. For this reason, it occurs that pulses in the third location *chě* are weak in men, and in women are firm (generally speaking), for if the opposite happens, a man follow a woman's pulse, and a woman a man's.

Commentary: Pulses either point toward radical wetness or primordial heat; or they are nature in their paths, or preternatural. Why do women and men have their own particular constitution? Because (according to the Chinese), the man who first appeared in the nature of thing is believe to have come into existence at the hour of *ym*, over which primordial head holds sway, and has a stronger quality. But woman came into existence at the hour of *Xin*, over which radical wetness holds sway, whose character is weaker. But now, three paths of primordial heat start their motion at the first location, and three paths of radical wetness start at the third location. Thus it happens that the pulses in a man are stronger in the first location, and pulses in a woman are stronger in the third location; on the other hand, in the third location, the pulses are weaker in a man and are stronger in a woman than in the first location, excepting many other reasons that the Chinese put forward.

Text: How does disease occur in a man? If a man has a woman's pulses (which are deficient), they indicate that the disease is further on the inside: at the right hand, if the pulse is at the right hand, and at the left, if the pulse is at the left. But if a woman has a man's pulses (which are surpassing) the disease is in the organs, and if the pulses are on the right or left, the disease will follow suit.

The Author Kipeus says: The pulses which do not observe but destroy the qualities of the four seasons of the year are either deficient or surpassing. Speaking about deficient ones, they arise due to the fact that that there is little radical wetness that holds sway over the bones and makes them heavy by refilling them. Such pulses are very highly deficient. But if you notice someone drinking and eating too little, and always less and less, know that their boy is wasting, and is in some way diminishing. The pulses that indicate this are called deficient from the targeted end; but if you see a person going to sleep and resting, but not evacuating;[234] and their eyes or ears are not functioning correctly, the pulses indicating this are called pulses of a deficient body. If you then notice that exhalation and inhalation do not agree with each other, and that five colors are destroying vibrancy in the body, the pulses which are then found are called pulse of a deficient soul. Finally, if you find that pulses of the four parts of the body (meaning the two feet, the same number of hands, and whatever things are connected to them) are disturbed, they are and are called pulses of deficient spirits.

Apart from these, there are some exceedingly deficient pulses over the course of thirty years (that is, they indicate that life will only be taken away in the thirtieth year); other pulses are deficient in a middling way, over the course of twenty years (that is, they indicate that life will end in the twentieth year); other

---

[234] *egerere*, literally, "to carry out," but it looks like it can be used of vomiting.

pulses are barely deficient, or very weakly so, over the course of ten years (that is, they indicate that life will be snatched after in the tenth year). Know that these pulses that we have discussed are found in the spring, summer, autumn, and winter. For this reason, if a person with a tall body is healthy and has a short pulse, know that that person's pulses are of the first sort, which are very deficient.

If a person is of a short stature and has long pulses, know that that person's pulses are of the second sort, which are less deficient, and promise a life of a lesser or middling time (that is, of twenty years). If that person has thin feet and hands, their pulses must be said to be of the third sort, which are very hardly deficient, promise life of a short number of years (namely, ten years). But if you notice that someone is deficient in their breathing and in the perfection of their spirits, understand that that person cannot typically live for much longer.

If there are short *tuon* pulses in a man's left hand, and in the right hand are long *cham* pulses, they indicate that those pulses are of deficient primordial heat, and they promise a life of only half a year. But if the pulses in a woman's right hand are short, and long in the left hand, they indicate that the pulses are of deficient radical wetness, promising that the woman's life will only be six months.

Beyond these enumerated deficient pulses, there are others, which we shall discuss below. There will be a discussion at some length on the change of the four seasons of the year, so that when, for instance, a spring-time pulse, which is in the location of the path of the liver (that is, it is in the second point of the left hand), gains a pulse of the path of the stomach, and is called the deficient pulse of the stomach. And because the heart-pulse should be at the first location in the summer, if the pulses of the path of the bladder or lungs appears, they are called deficient pulses of the bladder or lungs. If, in the autumn, pulses of the lungs ought to be seen in the first location of the right hand, but if they appear to belong to the liver or heart, they are called deficient pulses of the liver or heart. In the winter, if pulses of the path of the bladder or kidneys appear contained in the third location of the left hand, but on the other hand, if the pulses there appear to belong to paths of the heart or stomach, they are called deficient pulses of the heart or stomach. All of these things should be carefully noted, to see whether pulses are stopped at the first location *cum keu*, or after it. Because if there is no pulse in the first location, but there are some in the third location, like taut strings, those pulses have still the stomach's spirits. But if the upper and lower regions have no pulses, they indicate death. If either region is entirely without pulses, they indicate that a person is still alive.

*And those are the deficient pulses*

The signs of surpassing pulses are when someone has a particularly deep voice, and, when looking at things that are not too far away, everything is jumbled up and confused, as though one thing were something else.[235] These are called surpassing pulses, or pulses of a deficient mind.[236] If the body is obese and large and takes in a great deal of food and drink, the pulses that are then found belong to a person pondering many things anxiously; they are called surpassing, and if they talk nonsense and seem to walk about not only on their feet, but even on their hands, they are called surpassing pulses of a deficient body. And if they have the color of grasses, the surpassing pulses that then result are said to belong to a deficient soul. If you see thin or small pulses, that exhalation and inhalation do not correspond to one another (even if one is great), it is understood that these are among the surpassing pulses. And these are their indications, handed down to posterity from Emperor Hoamti, the most ancient of Doctors.

But let us consider the signs of the interpolation of pulses.

---

[235] *quasi unum quid esset*, literally, "as if one thing were something."
[236] *animi*, related to *anima* ("breath of life," "soul"). It generally refers to the "rational soul" (what we would call the "intellect"), but given the layers of translation here, the exact meaning is unclear.

Text: A person whose pulse gives a beat once and ceases in the second turn, will die on the next[237] day.

Commentary: Another book has: after one day, he dies.

Text: A pulse of two beats, which even afterwards stops once and is interrupted, indicates death on the third day.

A pulse giving three beats, and afterwards sitting still, shows death on the fourth day, and sometimes the fifth.

One giving four beats, and afterwards sitting still, indicates death on the sixth day.

One giving five beats, and afterwards sitting still once, indicates death on the fifth day, and sometimes the seventh.

A pulse giving six beats, then sitting still, indicates death on the eighth day.

One giving seven beats, and then sitting still, indicates death on the ninth day.

One giving eight beats and then sitting still indicates death on the tenth day.

A pulse giving nine beats and then sitting still indicates death on the tenth day, and sometimes on the eleventh day.

Commentary: Another book has: It also indicates death on the eleventh day, and that at the beginning of spring.

A pulse giving ten beats and afterwards sitting still indicates death at the beginning of summer.

(Commentary: Another book has: he dies at the beginning of spring.)

---

[237] *altera die*, literally, "on the other day."

A pulse giving eleven beats and afterwards sitting still, means the person will die on the summer solstice[238]

(Commentary: Another book has at the beginning of summer, and yet another, at the beginning of autumn.)

A pulse giving twelve or thirteen beats, and afterwards sitting still, means the person will die at the beginning of autumn.

(Commentary: Another book has, at the beginning of winter.)

A pulse giving fourteen or fifteen beats, and afterwards sitting still once, means the person will die at the beginning of winter.

(Commentary: One book has, at the beginning of the next summer.)

A pulse giving twenty beats and afterwards sitting still indicates death after one year, which will happen at the beginning of autumn.

A pulse of twenty-one beats, which afterwards sits still, indicates death after two years.

A pulse of 25 beats, which afterwards sits still, means the person will die at the beginning of winter. (Commentary: Another book has, he dies after one year, and sometimes two.)

A pulse of 30 beats, which afterwards sits still once, means the person will die after two years, and sometimes after three.

A pulse of 35 beats, which afterwards sits still once, means the person will die after the third year.

A pulse of 40 beats, which afterwards sits still once, means the person will die after the fourth year.

---

[238] The sentence is very compressed; technically, the Latin says that the pulse dies (*Pulsus...moritur*, without any subordination), but I think it's just a short-hand way to get the point across, or attempting to capture the nature of the original Chinese.

A pulse of fifty beats, which afterwards sits still once, means the person will die after the fifth year.

Pulses coming and going without interpolation, rest, and cessation, so that they do not break fifty beats, show that all organs and intestines have spirits, and for that reason are free from disease.

Commentary: *Sien kiñ san*, the aforementioned book, says: The spirits of the five Elements make up numbers of absolute[239] radical wetness and primordial heat, and at the same time they reveal that blood and spirits, coming and going by their own motion, travel through the paths of the pulses, and traverse them over the course of a night and a day.

A pulse coming from forty turns, which afterwards stands still once, shows that one organ is deprives of spirits, and thus that death is going to come after the fourth year, at the time in spring when grasses sprout.

A pulse coming from thirty turns, which afterwards stands still once, shows that two organs are without spirits, and so that death is going to come after three years, at the time that wheat ripens.

A pulse coming from twenty turns, which afterwards stands still once, shows that three organs are without spirits, and so death will come after two years, at the time when the fruit of the mulberry tree ripens and grows red.

A pulse coming from ten turns, and which then stands still once, shows that four organs are without spirits, and that death will come within the span of half a year. And if he avoids its, when the time *ci in mi in* comes (which time means "changes of more perfect brightness, and is the time around the second moon,[240] as the Chinese year starts with the first moon, which is around the beginning of February), the person will die. If they also make it

---

[239] Could also modify "spirits."

[240] *secundam lunam*, literally, "second moon," but seems to be an idiom referring to the number of days after a new moon.

past this time, death will not be able to be delayed for too terribly long, for at the following time of change, called *kŏ yn*, which means rain of the cornfields[241] and occurs around the third moon.

A pulse coming from five beats, and then cease, it indicates that five organs are without spirits, and thus that death will come after five days.

Then, if you see that the beat of one pulse hesitates and tarries for a long time, know that there is a strong disease in the heart, and occupies the middle part of it. If you see that two beats of two pulses are similarly hesitate drawing out their pause, know that there is a disease in the liver, and it occupies the outermost parts of it. If you notice that three pulse-beats are hesitating for too long, know that there is a disease in the stomach, and it resides in the middle of its lowest part. If you detect four pulse-beats tarrying too long, know that there is a disease in the bladder or kidneys. If you sense five pulse-beats tarrying too long, know that there is a disease in the extremities of the lungs.

If a sick person with a delicate or obese body has the five pulses that were just mentioned, they necessarily must die, and no medicine will benefit them. If a sick person should be possessed of a moderately full frame, the spirits of the aforementioned pulses can be adjusted.

First, it follows (based on this chapter and those that came before) what measure of time is necessary for pulses, and why the Chinese observe it so studiously. But pay very careful attention—through the pulses which you shall find in the third location, whether they are natural or preternatural, it indicates the condition of the third region of the body; through those that you will find in the first location *cun kĕu*, it indicates the condition of the uppermost region of the body; and through those that you will find in the middle or second pulse-location, it indicates the condition of the middle region of the body. In that middle location, if the pulses are tending towards primordial

---

[241] *segetum pluviam*, exact meaning unclear.

heat, they reveal the first region of the body, from navel to head; but if the pulses are tending towards radical wetness, they reveal the condition of the lowest portion of the body, from the navel to the feet. But when it happens that no pulses are found in the first location, it then happens that pulses of the third location do not advance to the middle location, because radical wetness is destroyed and deficient, since death must necessarily follow after radical wetness is destroyed and primordial heat appears weak. Understand then, that three pulse-locations, whether they have any pulses or not, indicate cold in the stomach, which is the reason why pulses arrive and pulse less. Therefore, the first location *cun keu* (which has a pulse) and the third location (which lacks it) indicates that a person absolutely will vomit, and if they do not vomit, they will die. If the first location is without a pulse and the third has a pulse, although it may be a difficult disease to cure, it gives a hope of life, just like a root, which still thrives (even after its branches are stripped bare) and promises fruit. If the pulse that should belong to a healthy person is detected and it still happens that this person dies, then it happens that the paths of the spirits are refilled in the bladder or the kidneys (sometimes in the gate of life) and are completely intercepted.

Secondly, it follows, based on what the cause of life is and where it resides, and how it is propagated throughout the body its perfection and deficiency are recognized through the pulses. But after we assign pulse locations and we demonstrate both the moveable part[242] and measure of the motion (which is their[243] cause) (and that motion begins and ends in that measure), it remains for us to deal with the pulses themselves and their nature; then we will produce and define the types of pulses such as are put forward by the Chinese; and we will also express them to the very imagination by pictures that they use for that purpose, as we find in the ancients and more modern writers; next, we will describe the six ordinary, or natural pulses (with three

---

[242] *mobile*

[243] *Illorum,* "of those things," point of reference unclear, probably in reference to pulse-locations here.

location in the right hand and three locations in the left—that is, the six fonts of life, meaning the organs and intestines); and afterwards, we will look into whether those same pulses continue on connaturally, or whether they change according to a variation in their properties over the four seasons of the year; and we will expose the harmful pulses that creep their way in, running contrary to what is natural, over the four seasons of the year; likewise, we will show how the symptoms of every disease can be diagnosed and predicted by pulses, as well how the Chinese reach their conclusions by colors, the sound of the voice, appetite, dreams, and other signs; and we will, if time permits, deal with diseases, fevers, and death itself; and we will note the practice of all this; at last, we will relate the reasoning used by the Chinese in practicing medicine.

Michal Boym

## CHAPTER SIXTEEN - A[244]

*The types of pulses that the Chinese assign (described also in images); likewise, the elements and four seasons of the year that hold sway over them, and what organ or intestine they gain their nature from.*

We have shown above that primordial heat and radical wetness (harmoniously and appropriately combined) give life and distribute it to the entire body, by force of the motion of blood and spirits; and the pulses that arise from this motion indicate either good or bad health in the designated hand-locations. Given this, let us undertake to deal with pulses. It is necessary to state that they have the nature of the motion and mobility from which they come. For this reason, since it is a threefold motion (according to the threefold path of primordial heat), and again, another threefold motion according to the threefold path of radical wetness, it follows that pulses, whichever motion they come from, whether connatural or preternatural, tend some towards primordial heat and some towards radical wetness. Likewise, because those two qualities variously include elements and their virtues in their various origins, that various pulses also tend towards various elements. Finally, because they begin in paths (or at least creep into paths), they should have the nature of those sources whose virtues they have a greater share of.

Now, to begin, we will provide a description of all pulses (which you will find expressed elsewhere in their own images), whether they aim at *yâm* or *iñ* (and they have the nature of that Element, and thus its source — that is, the organ and intestine). We will also provide the name. Below, we will discuss how someone can determine the diseases, symptoms, and affections of any part of the body, according to the individual pulses in six pulse locations that have been covered.

---

[244] There are two chapters with the title of "CAPUT DECIMUM SEXTUM" in the latin text.

The commonly received types of pulses are as follows: *Mĕ ciĕ piáo*, seven <pulses> which are on the outside; *me chum pa*, eight which are on the inside; then *kieŭ tao mĕ*, the pulses of nine paths; afterwards there are eight pulses *ki kīm pă mĕ* of extraordinary paths; finally, there are the pulses *quay mĕ*, seventeen monstrous pulses that are all fatal.

A description of the seven pulses which appear outside and tend towards *yâm*, primordial heat.

1. *Feu*: pulses floating on the surface tend towards *yâm*. The beat which one takes by finger seems deficient deep down,[245] superabundant at the surface. If you take it over and over, it will seem as though it is *tai quo*, a tremendously surpassing pulse.

Commentary: That this pulse appears deficient deep down comes from *in*, radical wetness; that an elevated pulse has a surplus comes from *yâm*, tremendously surpassing primordial heat. A very ancient book describes this pulse: The pulse *feŭ* clearly makes such a motion as is made by the leaf of onions,[246] when, although pressed down, it brings itself up.[247]

It is subject to the Chinese Element *kiñ*, that of metals.

When found in diseases, it indicates wind of the lungs.

2. The *keu* pulse tends towards *yâm*. Taking it by finger, one finds the beat floating even more, in both extremes; but in the middle, broken and empty. Thus, this pulse is not whole.

Commentary: The fire of primordial heat takes the pulse and makes it float. When it is floating, because it is without power, it is empty in the middle and full in the two extremities.[248]

---

[245] *deorsum*, means "down" (as in motion or locality), but here, in contrast with *ad superficiem*, I think it means "deep down"
[246] *folium ceparum*, literally "leaf of onions," maybe means "the rings of an onion"?
[247] Meaning uncertain.
[248] Meaning uncertain.

Michal Boym

A very ancient book says: A *keŭ* pulse has two heads, but is empty in their center.

It is subject to the Element of fire; when found in diseases, it indicates an abundance and emptying of blood.

3. *Hiě*, the sharp and close pulse, tends towards *yâm*. Taking it by finger reveals it in three locations in the hands. Its touch seems to be of such a sort as comes from a round gem moving down; and if you touch the location again, the beat seems to be falling, and one that neither enters or departs.

Commentary: The *hiě* pulse has the watery nature of primordial heat. A very ancient book says, the *hiě* pulse seems to be like the motion of a gem, which draws near and retreats, and is keen or sharp at the end. It is subject to the Element of water; when found in diseases, it indicates vomit, which wind opposes.

4. *Xě*: A full and solid pulse, it tends towards *yâm*. Fingers find its beat full; <it is a pulse> which, when it is elevated, has surplus.

Commentary: The pulse is full of the fire of primordial heat. The same book says, the full pulse seems to float in the middle.

Another ancient book says, the full pulse is identical with the long. It is subject to the Element of fire; when found in diseases, it indicates that the heart's heat is being suffocated.

5. *Hiên*. This is the pulse of the extended chord, it tends towards *yâm*. Whoever takes that pulse perceives that it is insufficient deep down, but when elevated, is surpassing.

It is like the beat of a bent bow; sometimes it is repeated. An ancient book says the same thing.

It is subject to the Chinese Element of the trees, or air; when found in diseases, it indicates pain in the eyes and exhaustion of the nerves.

6. *Kiù*, a vehement, intense, and strong pulse, tends towards *yâm*. A finger taking it in three locations in the hands finds that it is surpassing; and, when it is elevated, very fast. It is like the intense course of a torrent.[249]

The book says: the *kin* pulse is said to be like a taut string. It is subject to the Element of trees or air; when found in diseases, it indicates that wind is in control, and that pain arises from that.

7. *Kum*, the overflowing pulse, tends towards *yâm*. Whoever takes that pulse discovers that it is very great underneath, and is surpassing when it is elevated.

The book has: When it is elevated, it is surpassing, and is very great. It is subject to the Element of fire. When found in diseases, it indicates that heat is in control, and that there is pain in the head.

The eight types of pulses that are towards the inside, and tend towards *in*, radical wetness.

1. *Vi*, the small pulse, tends towards *iñ*. It is a beat which, when it is sought, draws near and retreats very weakly; and when sought over and over, it sometimes seems to exist, sometimes not.

Commentary: The rule of the small pulse is: that beat which tends to occur in autumn and winter arises from radical wetness.

The ancient book says the same thing: "The small pulse is subtle, exactly as if someone were feeling a thread of silk. It is subject to the Element of earth; when found in diseases, it indicates thick and corrupted blood, and thus, blood that is flowing downwards. It also indicates sorrow because of the surplus of wetness and the deficiency of heat.

2. *Xin*, the deep pulse, tends towards *in*. When the beat is sought, it seems to be found deep down; but when it is elevated, it

---

[249] Meaning unclear

completely fails to appear. When remiss, it travels through three pulse-locations and is perceived like soft cotton.

Commentary: The deep pulse comes from watery radical wetness, touches the nerves, rests upon the bones, is created properly from the deficient and opposing spirits of radical wetness, and excludes the spirits of primordial heat.

The book says the same: The profound pulse has a feel like soft cotton; it is found very near to the bones; it is subject to the Element of water; in diseases, it indicates a quantity of cold spirits.

3. *Huǒn*, that is, the remiss pulse, tends towards *iñ*. When the beat draws near and retreats, it is slow and sluggish, and the pulse consists of a not-great and slow part, and is called remiss.

Commentary: It comes from great heat, when wind damages the motion of blood and spirits, which thus cannot travel through each other in return.

The book says: The pulse is remiss when a small and slow pulse draws near and retreats gradually. It is subject to the Element of earth. When found in diseases, it indicates heat and rotten tepidity.

4. *Ci*, dull and thin,[250] tends towards *iñ*. Taking it by finger, it seems to be on the inside; but when it is elevated, it is not detected. It is empty at the beginning, but full at the end, which then shortly vanishes and is hard to find because of its subtlety.

Commentary: It is such because blood is more often damaged.

The book says, "The *ci* pulse seems to be similar to when someone scrapes the surface of cork[251] with a knife. It is subject to the Element of metals. In diseases, it indicates that the blood has been corrupted by radical wetness, and in a pregnant woman,

---

[250] *obtuso-rarus*

[251] *corticum*, from *cortex*, literally, "hull" or "shell," but often used of cork-bark, and thus cork.

that birth is imminent, and if the person does not have a womb, that their blood is corrupted."

5. *Chi*, the slow pulse, tends towards *iñ*. Only a finger applied strongly to the hand can find it, for it is rather hidden.

Commentary: It originates because an abundance of heat is weakened; thus, the motion of spirits and blood is condensing, and seems to be almost congealed.[252] Thus it is called the slow pulse, and is generally one that has only three beats over the course of one breath.

The book has the same.

It is subject to the Element of earth; when found in diseases, it indicates that spirits (air) is being created by the cold.

6. *Siú*: the gentle, floating, subtlest, softest, and weakest pulse. One may take it by hand only if it is touched <by cotton in water>.[253]

It tends towards *iñ*. Fairly often, it draws near and retreats, and will suddenly deceive the person taking it.

The book says: When it is found, it seems to go away immediately. It is subject to the Element of water.

In diseases, it indicates in particular the lower, cold part of the body.

7. *Fo*, the falling pulse, tends towards *iñ*. It seems to be perceived, but it hardly appears over the course of one breath. When sought over and over, it reveals itself, and it is not far removed from the three pulse locations.

---

[252] *congelatus*, literally, "frozen."
[253] *si tangeretur a gossypio intra aquam*, literally, "if it were touched from cotton within water."

Commentary: You will only find it after a diligent search. Its extremity—that is, its end, is not far from the pulse location *cuñ, quan, chĕ*.

The book says: It is a beat like a sunken object that soon emerges. When a strong touch is applied to the bones, sometimes it reveals itself. It does not have a picture, <but rather, the letter *miĕ*>[254], which means to seek.

It is subject to the Element of the trees, or air. In diseases, it indicates a conjunction and abundance of poisonous spirits.

8. *Jŏ*, the weak or fragile pulse, tends towards *iñ*. A finger takin it feels something like spun wool or cotton. It is perceptible with a very light touch; pressing down hard or strong makes it disappear.

Commentary: At the skin or flesh, it appears very gentle; the book says the same. It is subject to the Element of metals. In diseases, it indicates wind grouped together with spirits.

Notice 1: The pulses *hieu* and *kin*, those of the extended and intense chord; *vi* and *jo*, small and weak; *hiĕ* and *siŭ*, thick and gently floating; *feu* and *kúm*, floating and overflowing; *chi* and *ci*, slow and thin; *chin* and *fo*, deep and falling—<these pairs> seem to be very similar, even exactly the same, and for this reason, they indicate similar diseases, and finally, altogether different ones. Then, the pulses *feu* and *chin*, floating and deep; *kúm* and *ci*, overflowing (dense) and subtle; *hien* and *huēn*, intense and remiss; *sú* and *chi*, regular (excited) and slow; *Xe* and *hiu*, full and empty; ham and tuon, that of the extended chord (great) and small, Hie and ci are repeated and rare: Hien and vi pulses are completely opposite and at odds with each other, and indicate opposite diseases.

Notice 2: The seven pulses on the outside, which tend towards *yâm*, are generally perceptible in the pulse location of the left hand, because most of them there at the location of connatural

---

[254] Referring to Chinese characters?

pulses sneak their way in like guests, and they do so according to the changes in the human body, which are the causes of these sorts of pulses. Then, the eight pulses on the inside that correspond to *iñ* primarily tend to be perceptible in the right-hand pulse-locations, and that is because they make their way to the same place, the connatural pulse-location, in a similar manner, according to the changes of the body, as indicated above. The three left-hand pulse locations—*cuñ, quañ, chĕ*—experience changing of the pulses that happens to them—and they are called either *ueñ*, "tepid," or *fúm*, "windy," or *hañ*, "cold." These three things cause disease on the outside. At the other three right-hand locations, they experience changes of pulses according to the mastery of *caŏ*, the burnt qualities; *xe*, the wet qualities; *xu*, great billowing;[255] for these three things cause diseases on the inside. Take note of that with all due diligence, so you may understand the quality of diseases. Just as there are changes, the pulses sometimes seem to make their way to the right hand (from the seven exterior ones) and sometimes to the left (from the inside). Sometimes, radical wetness and primordial head attack each other and take them over (which is discovered from the pulses that have their nature; sometimes they suffocate each other by turns and sink, sometimes one pulse (or rather, one pulse's location) undergoes ten different changes. Indeed, since an account of the pulses is very subtle, it cannot be described here briefly. But because it is absolutely necessary to make note of it; because all the pulses have either *yâm* or *iñ* nature, and the qualities of the five Elements. But since seven and eight pulses make 15, but the elements are five, it follows that three pulses should be attributed to each Element. Thus, the pulse *feú ci*—floating, dull-and-thin, weak—have the nature of the Element of metals, so on concerning what has been already discussed.

So too you will understand that each individual related pulse, making its way into the six pulse-locations, has its own heaviness or lightness, just as the Elements whose nature they

---

[255] *aestus*, by extension, "fire," "heat" (different from *calor primigenius*, "primordial heat")

follow are heavy or light; or because of the fact that, out of the pulse locations, they hold the upper or lower location. As for the five Elements themselves, they repeatedly have and maintain an equality amongst themselves, and they repeatedly endure inequality, which can easily be detected in diseases. It also should be said that those things that are on the inside injure themselves, but they do not do mischief to themselves;[256] but those that move in turns on the outside, if you do not know those two things, you will be able to make a terrible mistake distinguishing the middle between heaven and earth, and the motions of the six spirits (for the body of man is like a small heaven and earth).

Harm on the outside creeps in, causes disturbance, and follows an evil nature: for instance, wind and radical wetness causing disturbances on the outside indicate that the Element of trees and fire (meaning the liber and heart) are suffering a terrible excess; and earth and metals (meaning the stomach and lungs) are deficient. Thus it is revealed that water (meaning the bladder) is insufficient to harmonize or restore them. This is as I said above, that harm, coming and moving on the outside (for instance, fire—that is, the heart—makes other Elements—that is, the organs—to ruin their own property. I have also said that those that reside on the inside do harm to themselves (that is, those same five elements—that is, the organs—cannot restore equality to themselves of their own accord). Therefore, it proves valuable to know well the nature and properties of Metals, Water, Trees (Air), Fire, and Earth—that is, the organs that share in their nature—and then to examine those that are empty and worn out, and those that are full and abundant. Furthermore, there is the damage of robbery,[257] the damage of thinness, and the damage that comes from the thing itself, which will be discussed below.

---

[256] *laedant* (literally, "hurt," "wound," "injure") vs. *faciunt malum* (literally, "do evil")

[257] *latrocinium*, literally, "brigandage," "highway robbery," "piracy;" from *latro*, "brigand," "highway robber"

It will further prove valuable to distinguish *feú, chám,* and *xín,* the surface, middle, and deep pulses for each location in the hand; to carefully examine the locations and pulses that are there, to see whether they agree and are harmonious with the nature of the locations (that is, to see whether those paths which were assigned to the aforementioned pulse-locations agree with the nature and qualities of the pulses that otherwise approach almost like guests, or else sneak their way in).

If they do not correspond, you should know that they are strangers and guests, as they say, and are preternatural. If you clearly see this, it will be easy to recognize what those things are that cause damage on the inside, and what they are that move on the outside; what the diseases are that appear on the outside like leaves, and what ones start on the inside, like roots.

Notice 3: Doctors first assigned seven pulses to the outside, eight to the inside, which in total are fifteen, such that they can be used to determine sufficiently the condition, life, and death of organs and intestines. But after they had recognized that other pulses also held sway throughout the year (for, just as the heavens have twenty-four changes of the air, so is it is in the human body, into which the heavens flow in particular), they found twenty-four different pulses—or rather, they added nine pulse-paths to those fifteen. But I would think that these new pulses added properties to the ones that have been related, rather than creating new pulses.

The pulses of the nine paths are called *kieù táo inè*

First: *Chaṁ*, that is, the long pulse, tends towards *yâm*. The beat in three pulse locations, like a shaking lance, when it is elevated, has surplus. It is also called long when it departs from its typical location; a very ancient book says the same. It originates from the path of the large intestines; when in diseases, it indicates that the body is feverish and deeply troubled.

Second: *tuon*, the short pulse, tends towards *iñ*, is deficient, and does not reach its typical location. The book says: "It does not reach to the middle of the finger. It comes from the stomach. In diseases, it indicates that the hands and feet are sweating, and that food is not being digested. It is akin to the motion of a grain of rice."

Third: *hiú*, the empty pulse, tends towards *iñ*. Its beat is not sufficient, and when it is elevated, it does not reach.

Commentary: It is not full, from a depletion of blood.

The ancient book has: "When it is elevated, even when sought, it is deficient. It begins in the path of the heat; it is similar to a ball of silk threat. In diseases, it indicates fear, weak power, and difficult breathing.

Fourth: *Sú*, the swift or not-wide pulse (tight and swift),[258] tends towards *yâm*. Its beat is fast, and takes root in the first location *cuɱ keu*, where, if it increases, it promises death; but if it gathers internally and somewhat hides away, it promises life.

Commentary: The pulse that comes very frequently, and sometimes sits still for one turn, and comes again, is called swift. It starts from natural heat, which comes from the path of the bladder, or kidneys. In diseases, it indicates that the *yâm* and *iñ* are very troubled.

Fifth: *Kiè*, the bound or interrupted pulse, tends towards *iñ*. The beat is sometimes approaching, sometimes departing or returning.

Commentary: The pulse is frequent, and coming almost one atop the other; and afterwards sitting still and returning.

The book says: When a pulse comes that is wide, sitting still, and returning, it is called *kiě*. It begins with the path of the lungs. In diseases, it indicates that the assembled spirits, sorrow, and weariness are hidden in the stomach.

---

[258] *arcto-celer*

Sixth: *tái*, "the overseer," is called the pulse of death, the killing pulse;[259] it tends towards *iñ*; it moves, and in returning, it strives to elevate itself over and over, and it cannot elevate itself. It is formed from its return and its condition (rest). When taking it, one notices that it elevates itself forceful at some point.

The book says: This pulse, as it comes, sits in the middle and cannot go back. It begins with the soul and the body. In diseases, it indicates that the spirits are dissipated, the organs and intestines are destroyed, and that death approaches.

Seventh: *Kieū*, that is, the dragging pulse, tends towards *iñ*. If you take it only in the typical manner, it will not be perceptible; but it will be perceptible if you look for it by pressing your finger down rather strongly.

The book says: "If it is sought, it is not found fully unless you press forcefully."

Commentary: It is fairly hard and deep, and has power, and it does not change. It originates in the path of the liver. In diseases, it indicates pain in the bones and wandering upward of spirits.

Eighth: *tum*, "moved." The pulse of motion tends towards *iñ*. It can be taken by the finger, but whenever it should be elevated, it vanishes. It is found when looked for over and over and is not far from its proper place.

Commentary: The pulse of motion is said to be neither approaching nor retreating. This pulse seems (since it neither comes near nor goes away, but is constant) like a very swift motion; but one which, because of the speed with which it travels about, seems not to move, and is like a resting mountain. This pulse is called (since it neither comes near, nor goes away, but is constant), as the put it, "orbicular."

The book says: "If you cast a millstone into the water, this pulse is very similar to the motion that is made by that action in still

---

[259] *intercidens*,could be from *intercido*, "die," or *intercido*, "kill." Something like "falling / felling"

water. It originates in the path of the small intestines. It indicates that all the organs are exhausted, and corrupted blood is moving downward."

Ninth: *Si*, the subtle pulse, tends towards *iñ*. The beat feels like cotton to the touch, approaching and retreating, very small. It begins in the path of the navel. In diseases, it indicates that the bladder is lacking the marrow's nourishment; that col, a deficiency of power, is troubling the inner regions and flowing down.

*Kí kīm pa mě*, the order of the pulse of extraordinary paths Twelve paths have fifteen streams, and these streams ultimately derive from the twelve paths. They are connected to the paths, and apart from the twelve streams which correspond to the twelve paths, it is possible to find three other streams: <the path> of great primordial heat in the hands, running from the large intestine, has a stream of the same name, *lo*, and so on. But since it is not a thirteenth path, the *lo* stream is called *pi chi tá lo*, "the great stream from the spleen;" and the fourteenth is called *yn ki ào lo* the stream of the humid root to the heat *jám kiáo lo*, "the stream of primordial heat reaching to the same place."

But take note that although the pulses of these three streams belong to extraordinary[260] paths, in some fashion they are connected to the ordinary paths. But although pulses of other extraordinary paths trace their origin from ordinary paths, they do not follow them. These paths have eight pulses and eight locations, which also indicate various illnesses.

First: *yâm quêy*, the chain of primordial heat. The pulse-path lies at the confluence of all *yam* chains, which form a long circle (like a worm) around the head; and afterwards, it goes askew; when it rests in the mouth of the chest, it causes diseases, and sends primordial heat down to the stomach; and thus, at the heart, which takes on that damage, from which heat and cold move to the outside, there is a cold-and-hot[261] disease. The

---

[260] *extravagantium*, literally, "wandering outside."
[261] *frigido-calidus*

cause of the disease is that the chains of primordial heat rely upon ordinary paths but will not be connected with the body.

This pulse-location *yâm quêy* is in all locations where the *yâm* pulse-paths are found.

Second: *iñ quêy*, the chain of radical wetness. This pulse-path comes from the confluence of all the chains of radical wetness; it makes its way down and makes a course of the body like a worm. Its seat is in the middle of the chest, where it also causes disease, based on the fact that it suffocates all the paths of radical wetness and sends them down to the spleen, and then to the heart. Damage to this path comes from the path of diminished wetness for the feet.[262] The disease that arises from it wearies the heart and causes it pain, and it is on the inside in the blood, and not on the outside. The *iñ quêy* pulse-location is in all locations where pulses of the paths of radical wetness exist.

Disease coming both from *yâm quêy* and *iñ quêy* indicates that there is great internal distress, and that the nobleness of spirit[263] is destroyed, and the body is corrupted by sluggishness and laziness.

Third: *yâm kiáo*, the path of primordial head towards the heel. This pulse-path in the heel makes a circuit of the high bone in the heel; as it moves up, it reaches the head-location that is called *di fum xi ten* (the extremity of the hair). Its motion is like a snake, it resides in the belly.[264] The disease lies at the feet joints, where it creates a mass and robs it of power; in the heart, though, it causes fear. This path originates in the paths of radical wetness in the feet and hands.

Fourth: *iñ kiáo*, the path of radical wetness to the heel of the foot. The pulse and path make a circuit of the lofty mouth of the heel

---

[262] Literally, "the evil of this path is the path of diminished wetness of the feet."

[263] *animi genorositatem*

[264] *ventriculo*, possibly short for *ventriculus cordis*, "ventricle of the heart." It appears a few more times in the text.

on the side. It advances to the throat, and then to the eyes. The pulse is like an extended[265] chord; the disease that it causes occupies the hands and the feet and their connections,[266] and it takes away the power of walking, and also reduces the spirits of the intestines and nerves. It originates in the paths of defective radical wetness in the feet and hands.

Note: All the pulses that are full of radical wetness and are soon scattered approach the heel path of radical wetness, and they indicate that there is damage in the radical wetness, but not in heat. Thus, heat is remiss, and wetness is intense. Next, from the aforementioned intensity and remissness, depletion and refilling follow; and then *iñ kiâo*, the heel path of radical wetness, spinning around the mouth and making its way upward, creates a disease on the inside, which is also intense, but remiss on the outside. But *yâm kiâo* is a cold disease, and it resides in the *fum fú* location, for heat is carries on the outside (just as wetness betakes itself on the inside), so that, if it exists on the outside, it is necessary for the sick person to produce sweat; if on the inside, it is necessary to have an emetic.[267]

Fifth: *chŭm*, the transverse path, permeating the spirits in the great middle part of the body, from the path in the feet of pure heat. The location is above the navel, towards the middle of the belly. But its pulse is like the beat of bird gathering seeds, which climbs by making advances in the chest and is scattered

---

[265] *chordae extensae*. The verbs *tendo*, *extendo*, and *intendo* (and their participle forms, *tensa*, *extensa*, and *intensa*) are used repeatedly, although the meaning is not always clear. Literally, the verbs mean "stretch," "stretch out," and "stretch towards." Sometimes, in verbal forms, it means "points towards" or "tends towards." In participial form (as here) it seems to mean "stretched" or "taut" (especially modifying *chorda*, which often means a string on an instrument). The exact meaning of these forms may be unclear; in those cases, I tend to translate with cognates ("extended," "intended").

[266] *illis conjuncta*, "the things connected to them," maybe "joints"?

[267] *portionem purgativam*, literally, "a share for purging;" I think this may just be the equivalent for this period of "induce vomiting."

randomly to the sides.[268] Between the bladder (kidneys) and the third region of the body, where the aforementioned location is, the "city of spirits,"[269] (the spirits' workshop is there), perfection and irrigation are lost; thus, the four parts (meaning the hands and feet) are afflicted with a yellow mass.[270] It is subject to the path of radical wetness in the hands; it causes pain in the stomach to make its way inwards.

Sixth: *Gín me*, the pulse of a pregnant person, is a path in the middle of the navel, which descends to the bending twist, and to that which is below it. That pulse-path is without a head or beginning but has an extremity. Its course is around the belly,[271] and it reaches up to that location which is called the gate of winds. The disease belongs to women who are suffering diarrhea on the inside, and it robs the four parts (meaning the hands and feet) of power. It is subject to the path of great primordial heat, which sends this stream to the heart, which it wearies, and it reveals that weariness in the red color of the face and dryness of the mouth, and it even makes its way to the *quan uên* location; and from there, it comes to the throat.

If a woman has already conceived, she has this disease.

Seventh: *To me*, the governing pulse, as they call it. Its path is in the lowest location of the lowest part, towards the last orifice that climbs up towards the aforementioned *fum fu* head-location. The pulse is like an extended chord. The disease that it indicates is cause by an abundance of spirits; it brings sadness, pain in the sides, and darkness in the eyes. It is subject to the path of diminished radical wetness in the feet.

Eighth: *Tui*, <the path> of the girdle or belt. The pulse and its path are within the sides of the body; they make a circuit of the whole body. The pulse is like butterfly,[272] having a long tail;

---

[268] *ad latum utrinque*, literally, "to the side on both sides."
[269] *civitas spirituum*
[270] *tumore flavo*
[271] *ventriculum*
[272] *papilionis*

sometimes it pulses, sometimes it is still. It has mastery over the feet and hands, which it renders immobile. In the kidneys and bladder, it causes pain. It comes from the path of pure primordial heat in the feet; moreover, the stomach seems to be full, as though it is hiding water on the inside. Their disease is cold.

*Seventeen monstrous and mortal pulses*

First: *Chîa yên*, motion of the frog. This pulse is so called because it moves no differently than does a leaping frog. It advances through three pulse-location. Over the course of a whole breath, it never appears full, and only pulses once. By finger, it feels like leaping.[273] It indicates a malignant fever; and on the third day, death. But if it is perceptible in the location where the bladder or kidney location has been assigned, it indicates that death will come after a day. The pulse is called *Sanxi*, destroying the body. The codex says: The soul departs, and the body becomes a corpse.

Second: *Yû vî*, the tail of the fish. This pulse is so called because it moves the finger like a swimming fish, its tail unmoved. Sometimes it gives a beat, sometimes it sits still. It is perceptible over the course of one breath, and then a malignant fever suffocates wetness. Whoever has this pulse dies after two days, and if they are elderly, after half a day. It is called *kiue xi*, dividing the body. This pulse indicates that the bladder (kidneys) are being destroyed; it is just like when a fish moves it head without moving its tail. If you detect it in the morning, know[274] that whoever has it will die in the evening.

Third: *Yen tāo*, the hidden sword. This pulse is so called because (just as a sword hidden in the hand shakes suddenly) it appears and disappears quickly. The speed of that pulse is because, over the course of one exhalation <and inhalation>,[275] there are two

---

[273] *Digitus saltum percipit*, literally, "A finger senses leaping."

[274] *resolve*, literally, "loosen," here perhaps literally translated as "reveal!"

[275] *introspiratio*, I think this is a mis-print for *introspirationis*. The first option would have to be the (singular) subject of the sentence, but doesn't agree with the plural verb.

beats. It indicates that the lungs are being destroyed. The illness is one of the nostrils letting out blood. Whoever has such a pulse dies after two days; if the disease in the lungs is old, after one day. It is called *him xi*, <the pulse of> the walking corpse."

Fourth: *Feu liên*, the turned-out leaf of the flower call *liên* (*liên*[276] is a flower that produces a fruit like round almonds, which grow in laces). The beat reaches the hand with exactly this sort of figure—it is small at the outset; afterwards, at the end, it descends obliquely, and it is also unequal. It pulses once over the course of a whole breath. It indicates that the chest, being full of spirits, has a shortness of breath. In diseases, such a pulse indicates that old men will die after three days, youths after one day. It is called *sum xi*, <the pulse of> the corpse being carried outside.

Fifth: *Kem xam feu che*, that is: the fatty broth floating upwards, and giving off bubbles or little spheres like gems, swimming on the surface. The pulse is like that: when it comes, it is small; when it goes away, it is large. It indicates weak spirits.

It is called *hie* and *fu fec*, "boiling" and "bubbling water." Thus, over the course of a whole breath, it gives twelve beats, and sits still once. The ancient book says: By finger, a beat is perceptible, as though they were waves of swimming broth. Whoever has such a pulse in the morning may anticipate death in the evening. Appearing in the middle location, where the pulse-paths for the spleen and stomach are, it indicates death after three days. It is called *feu xi*, <the pulse of> the swimming corpse.

Sixth: *Chen keu*, the opening of the goblet. This pulse is so called because it feels to the finger like the shape of the aforementioned vessel, for one can feel two heads (or rather, lips), empty and deep, with a middle. When it goes away and comes near, it has a motion like a hand that is wrapped around a rope. Over the course of a whole breath, there are eight beats, and sometimes nine; and they indicate death after a day; and if they add one beat to those that were mentioned before above, it indicates death

---

[276] Looks like this probably means "lotus"

after one hour. They are called *kuem xi*, <the pulses of> the oiled corpse.

Seventh: *Cio chui*, the beat of birds or chickens when they gather grain with their beaks. These pulses are so-called <because>, when the come, they are fast, and prick the finger just as when a chicken gather grain. Sometimes, they make three beats over the course of a whole breath; sometimes eight or nine. All indicate death after three days—and if they are found in the pulse-location that is assigned to the path of the stomach, after one hour. It is called *su, xi*, <the pulse> arranging for the body. The ancient book says: The beats of eating chickens—constant and sometimes fast—indicate the stomach (the origin of spirits that are made from the substance of food) is deficient, and will be restored with difficulty.

Eighth: *Ilo leu*, that is, house-droplets.[277] This pulse, which is similar to running water (or rather, water dripping, drop by drop, off the house), generally has three beats and interrupts the course. You will find them over the course of a whole breath in sick people. When they come, they are full; when they depart, they are very weak. In old people, they indicate death after ten or thirty days; in youths, after three. Whoever has such a pulse in the location of the stomach-path dies after one day. They are called *pim xi*, "<the pulse of> the ailing corpse." The ancient book says: They indicate that the spirits of three heats are depleted and separated from the stomach. They are like drops of rain falling down from the roof.

Ninth: *Tan xe*, that is, the pulse of the stony ball.[278] It is so called because it has the beat which is made by throwing of a rock, or a ball game. It does not return again over the course of a whole breath. It indicates that the spirits of the path of diminished

---

[277] *domus stillicidium*, "droplets of the house," where *stillicidium* means "trickling water," but has a very specific meaning of "drops of water dripping off a house."

[278] *pilae lapideae; pila* can mean several things, including "mortar" (as in mortar and pestle), "column," and "ball" (as for throwing). The context makes it seem like the throwing ball, but it's unclear.

radical wetness in the feet, running from the bladder, is being destroyed. When it comes and goes, it makes the motion that someone blowing into a feather makes. Sometimes, its has a single beat over the course of a whole breath; other times, another single beat over two whole breaths. Both indicate death after a day. It is called *Xoen xi*, the soul of the corpse. The ancient book says: The beat that travels quickly an comes slowly indicates that life is being broken. It is like the motion that the throwing of a stone produces.

Tenth, *kiaj so*, a pulse very similar to the motion of an untied string. It is frequent and scattered, and it is not constant, or even connected, exactly like when someone has untied a string or belt from the body. Over the course of several breaths, it sometimes has a single pulse; when it comes, it soon scatters; when it goes away, it pauses, and its motion seems as if you were to twist plants in the manner of rope. It indicates death after the third day; and if it is found in the location of the bladder-path, after one day. It is called *tai xi*, <the pulse of> the corpse's belt.

Eleventh: *Siĕ kíum*, the roots of two plants thus called,[279] which vanish just as soon as they swim up. This pulse is similar to them; when it is taken by finger, it is found to be deficient; but when it is elevated, to be full. Nine or ten beats occur over the course of a whole breath; when the beats approach, they are long; when they go away, the lack power. If you see this pulse in the path of diminished radical wetness (the path of the bladder) in the feet, you will die after a day. It is called *fi xi*, <the pulse of> the flying corpse.

Twelfth: *Hú nón*, a globule or clod of earth. The pulse makes a beat similar to this. It is full and large to the touch, and has neither beginning nor end. It happens nine or ten times over the course of one breath. It indicates death after two days. If it is found in the location of the bladder's path, it indicates that one's

---

[279] *duarum herbarum sic dictarum radices*, maybe "so-called plants" or "the aforementioned plants"?

spirits are at their end, and death will come after one day. It is called *cive xi*, the pulse of the destroyed corpse.

Thirteenth: *Fan pai*, overturned and destructive. This pulse is like two small beans floating in water; its beat is like their motion. When it comes, it is light; when it goes away, it is slow. Over the course of one breath, it occurs seven or eight times, and it is present in malignant fever, when the sick person is delirious because of their toil. Whoever has such a pulse dies after one hour. It is called *te xi*, carrying away the corpse.

Fourteenth: *Ta ke*, the pole or axis. This pulse is like the pointer-finger. When the beat comes, it is large; when it goes away, it is full; it never stands still or rests; one beat occurs, sometimes over the course of a whole breath, sometimes two breaths, but it is very weak. Whoever has these pulses dies after an hour. This pulse is called *kien xi*, dragging the corpse.

Fifteenth: *Kiai so*, <the pulse of> loosening the loins. This pulse is like a very fine, very delicate threat. When it comes, it is small and without a head. It is like the motion of someone folding something up and not being able to go back again. It indicates that the original spirits are at an end. It makes ten beats over the course of one breath, and it subsides after them. It indicates death after a day. This pulse is called *Cŏ xi*, <the pulse of> the corpse's mourner.[280]

Sixteenth: *To Xi*, means, bringing on Death. This pulse is like the harp of a performer, with an intense beat. When it comes, it is very frequent; when it departs, it is less frequent. It has a great beginning and a very small end, like a struck harp. Over the course of a breath, there occurs either a single beat, or else three very fast ones without a pause, or else eight, with a subsequent pause.

They indicate death after a day. This pulse is called *mày xi*, the buried corpse.

---

[280] *deplorantis cadaver*, literally, "<a person> weeping over a corpse."
122

The aforementioned pulses are all fatal, and just as each one can be accurately determined over the course of a regular breath (which, as we mentioned, was is the measure for all pulses), one should also understand the same thing from the sick peoples' voice (or the sounds they make), their complexion and appetite. If you reach that point, you have reached perfection in the art, for then to you will be able to predict diseases and conditions and death.

## CHAPTER SIXTEEN - B[281]

*What the connatural pulses are in the three right-hand location, and in the three left-hand locations, assigned to the twelve paths and emanating from the organs and six intestines.*

Note first that, both in the right and left hand, the first location *cuñ keu*, is subordinate to *lao yâm*, perfect primordial heat; and, as for the distance, it occupies nine parts of *kieu fuèn* (a finger measure), out of the ten aforementioned *ki*—that is, an unequal number. But in both hands, the third or last location, *chĕ*, is subordinate to *lao iñ*, perfect radical wetness; and as for distance, it occupies ten part in an equal number (that is, one whole finger measure). Next, the middle location, or second pulse *quañ*, is the boundary that distinguishes the first and the third location, and combines primordial heat and radical wetness with each other; for the first location *cun keu* is the seat of primordial heat, and it should have a connatural pulse, swimming in nine parts; and the third location *chĕ* should have a connatural pulse of radical wetness in ten parts—that is, one joint *Xin seu* deep. But the middle or second location *quan* should have its seat in both, and a connatural pulse, neither above nor below the swimming <pulse>, but in the middle between those two. Since it originates in *quēy ki*, the spirits of the stomach (and it certain resides in the middle), so it indicates the disposition and equality of the first and third pulse-locations. If it loses this,[282] both the first and third pulse-locations indicate that heat and wetness are surpassing or deficient; and if they wander outside the boundaries of *yn ci* (the name of the location at the farthest part of the palm) and *chĕ* (the other location at the farthest part of the *chĕ* measure), and the middle pulse location *quan* appear with no spirits moderating them, it means that men that have such pulses will die without disease.

---

[281] There are two chapters with the title of "CAPUT DECIMUM SEXTUM" in the latin text.
[282] Seems like "this" must be *aequalitatem*, "equality" here.

Text: Some pulses are *tai que*, surpassing; others are *tu kie*, deficient; sometimes, *iñ* and *yâm* overpower one another; sometimes, the *feu* pulses turn back[283]; at other times, *iě* are surpassing; at still other times, they travel inside and outside their boundaries. Why? Because, when it moves to the middle location *quan yâm*, if the swimming pulse crosses beyond the nine parts of a finger-measure, the pulses are called *tai quo*, surpassing. If they do not reach them, they are called *pu kie*, deficient. Then, if they ascend the outermost location *iu ci* in the palm of the hand, they are called overflowing; whatever move beyond their boundaries and reach the inside, such pulses are said to belong to overwhelming radical wetness. But when it moves ahead of or beneath the middle location *quan*, towards radical wetness, the pulses are one whole joint's span deep, which are called surpassing if they move past that span; deficient if they do not reach it; and pulses are *feu*, retrocedent, if they do not reach the *che ce* location, because they approach the boundary and reverse course to the outside, and are called pulses of *yâm*, conquering primordial heat.

Commentary: Before the middle location in each hand, it is proper for the swimming pulses of primordial heat in the first location to move in nine parts (in an unequal number). After the second location (the middle), the third location of radical wetness, *chě*, should have deep pulses of a full span (ten parts *iñ*, with an even number). Both pulses indicate that the person is in good health, since those locations differentiate between *yâm* and *iñ*, which are kept in a joint union, from which equality and moderation comes. Thus it happens that one may never overwhelm the other. If one happens to overwhelm another, then the pulses are: *tai quo*, surpassing; *pu kie*, not reaching or deficient; *iě*, surpassing; *feu*, retrocedent; *quan*, encroaching upon territories or not reaching. When *iñ* spirits are in particularly great supply, they make *yâm* spirits not be able to move downward from the location where they come from, where

---

[283] *retrocedunt*, "yield back." Its participial form, *retrocedentes*, is used extensively in this section, and I try to translate it with the cognate "retrocedent."

it is necessary for them to travel from their proper location; and for the pulse to climb to the *in ci* location, where the pulses are that are called overflowing—because, of course, *vai quān* have advanced beyond their boundaries, and the *nŭy kie* have not been able to reach the inside; for a great deal of conquering radical wetness overwhelms primordial heat, for which reason the pulses of radical wetness are said to have *tăi quŏ*, surpassing <pulses>, and primordial heat has *pu kie*, deficient <pulses>. If spirits of primordial heat exceptionally numerous, they make the wetness move up along with its spirits and descend from their connatural location and wander below the fourth location *che ce*, where the pulses that one finds are called *feŭ*, retrocedent; that is, the *nŭy quan* advance within the actual boundaries, and the *vai kie* advance no further to the outside, for conquering primordial heat overwhelms radical wetness: the first one has deficient pulses, the latter surpassing.

Text: *feu*, retrocedent pulses; and *ye*, overflowing pulses, tend to be pulses of *chĕ cam̄*, the straight intestine. Whoever has them also dies with disease.

Commentary: Both indicate that heat and wetness are not sticking to each other, because one is separated from the other, they fall short of one another, since *yâm*, primordial heat, produces nothing, and nothing turns into radical wetness—thus, they are mutually mixed up with one another quite thoroughly. They produce *chĕ cam̄*, the pulse of the straight intestine, and since the stomach has no spirits through which it might return its heat and wetness to a moderate level, it occurs that, although a person may be without disease, because one is conquered by the other, the person will die soon.

## Model

| First, *cum* | | Second, *quañ* | Third location, *chĕ* | |
|---|---|---|---|---|
| The pulse and motion of *yâm*, primordial heat | | The boundary between both | The pulse and motion of *iñ*, radical wetness | |
| Whatever pulse enter the location *iñ ci* is overflowing, traveling beyond the boundary and sitting within it. It indicates that someone is liable to death. | Whatever pulse surpasses nine parts is called *tai quo*, surpassing, which does not reach *pu kiĕ*, deficient. It indicates illness. | Whatever pulses are in the *chum* location, which is *chĕ* deep, indicates a healthy person. | Whatever pulse surpasses *cum*, the span of a finger-measure, are *tai quo*, surpassing. Those which do not reach, are deficient. They indicate disease. | Those that enter the location *chĕ ce* are called retrocedent, regathered within the boundary and standing outside. They indicate that someone is liable to death. |

Whatever pulse floats on the top at nine parts *feu* indicates a health person

Note carefully that, in the three locations of both the left and right hand, if the pulses are connatural, they should be either swimming, or middling, or deep. If the *feu*, swimming pulses, degrade into *tai huo*, then they become surpassing, either *ta* (great), *cham* (long), *Xe* (full and solid), *hien* (like a taut string), *kúm* (overflowing), *keú* (flat in each extremity, and broken up in the middle), or *hie* (frequent). ut if a *chum* pulse degrades into *pa kie*, then they become deficient pulses, either *si* (subtle), *tuon* (short), or *hui* (empty), as well as *chi* (slow), *me* (weak), *fo* (moving inwards), or *chi* (thin).

Only *chum* pulses are in the middle of the belly (which indicate spirits); neither large nor subtle nor small (*pú ta pú si*); likewise, they are *pú cham pú taon*, neither long nor short; *pú chon pú feu*, neither deep nor floating at the surface; *pú kie pú kua*, neither deficient nor surpassing, or whatever is called by the same name. When taking a pulse by finger, one finds them moderate, and they can be called spirit-pulses for the stomach, because they are the mean between the two extreme pulses.

Second, note that connatural pulses, which correspond to the three locations in each hand and indicate a shared origin of their paths and conditions, have a general cause with primordial heat and radical wetness in the blood and spirits that are carried by that motion. But the distinction and quality of the pulses comes from the order and distinction of the threefold path of the same primordial heat and the threefold path of the same radical wetness. Just as they emanate from their sources in various ways (and the difference in the pulse is explained in the aforementioned locations) and the entire cause of the difference between the order and the connatural pulses is the heat and wetness in the three location of each hand; just as they share the inherent properties of their sources in the motion-paths of blood and spirits.

Text: Do pulses have the measure of radical wetness and primordial heat? They absolutely do, for *hú* exhalation leaves the heart and lungs; *hie* inhalation enters the bladder and liver, and these two form a whole *siě*, breath. The stomach, situated in the middle and receiving the taste its nourishment, has a pulse (by which its condition is indicated) also in the middle.

Commentary: Pulses have distinct and divergent spirits of radical wetness and primordial heat. Blowing out and blowing in,[284] as they call it is seen in exhalation and inhalation. The heart and lungs reside in the uppermost part; primordial heat, being predominate over their spirits, appears in the ejection of an exhalation. But the bladder and liver reside in the lower part, and being dominant over their spirits, <primordial heat> appears in the drawing in during inhalation. The spleen and stomach, although they do not pertain to the ejection or drawing in of a breath, nevertheless, because <primordial heat> holds sway over and controls the nourishment that is to be taken in (the substance of which forms spirits), just as it has a middle location among the organs, so is its disposition indicated in the middle of the pulses, and pulses are found as the mean between those pulses that occur over the course of inhalations and exhalations.

Text: The pulses floating at the surface comes from primordial heat; and deep pulses come from radical wetness. Thus, all tend towards either wetness or heat; but the heart and lungs are surface-floating pulses; so how does one tell them apart? As follows: if the pulses are *feu ta san*, swimming, great, those that also suddenly scatter, then they pertain to the heart and indicate its natural state; if, however, they are *feu tuon*, swimming, short, and thin, they pertain to the lungs and indicate *their* natural state. Likewise, the liver and bladder (kidneys) have a deep pulse. But how can they be distinguished? If the pulses are *Xin kin cham*, deep, strong, intense, and long, because these pertain to the liver, they indicate its natural disposition; but if they are *Xin so*, deep, weak, then they realize that they point to the bladder (kidneys) and their condition.

The stomach sits in the middle, like a guardian of the state; and thus, the pulses that indicate its condition are in the middle, and

---

[284] *Exsufflatio & insufflatio*

have the duty of moderating radical wetness and primordial heat in the other pulses.

Commentary: A great pulse that immediately scatters and is long, points to primordial heat. Pulses that are short, thin, intense, weak, and empty come from radical wetness. Because they are called *Xe*, stones, you should recognize that they are deep (for they seek the lowest they can, just like a stone). The pulses that climb up are called surface-floating; it is in their nature to be lifted up and sent off. Those that move down, though, are deep. It is in their nature be completely undetectable if taken gently by hand, and only to be found if pressed rather firmly. Then, since the heart and lungs sit over all the others, the pulses that indicate their condition should be surface-floating; and since the bladder and liver are downward, the pulses that indicate their condition should be deep.

Note carefully that great swimming pulses, and those that are soon scattered, because they come from *chîm yâm* (from most perfect primordial heat), thus they indicate the natural condition of the heart; and short and thin swimming pulses, which come from *yâm chúm chī iñ* (from radical wetness which is in the middle of primordial heat) indicate that a connatural character to the lungs. Deep, intense, and long pulses, because they come from *iñ chum chī yâm* (from primordial heat that is in the middle of radical wetness) indicate the natural condition of the liver; and deep, soft, and weak pulses, because they come from perfect radical wetness, <through radical wetness in the feet, with regard to perfect primordial heat>, it is understood not to be mixed, but simple. Then, through *yâm chúm chī iñ* and *iñ chum chī yâm*, understand "the heat within radical wetness" and "radical wetness within primordial heat," or that is, in the middle of primordial heat; but know that the equal mixing of the two (that is, heat and wetness) means the pulses of the stomach, which are subject to earthly properties. When it is actually in the middle of the lungs and bladder, even as it propagates through properties from the center to all the organs and bring moderation to their primordial heat and radical wetness, thus its pulses are in the middle of other pulses. A student should pay very close attention to these things.

Text: Some pulses are *yĕ yñ yĕ yâm*, coming from the one source of radical wetness and one source of heat; other are *yĕ iñ Ch yâm*, comes from one source of radical wetness and two of heat; others are *yĕ iñ sañ yâm*, coming from one source of radical wetness and three of heat. Next, there are *yĕ yâm yĕ iñ*, coming from one source of heat and one of wetness; others are *yĕ yâm Ch in*, coming from one source of heat and two sources of radical wetness; and still others comes from *yĕ yâm sañ iñ*, coming from one source of heat and three of radical wetness. Thus it follows that *cūn keu*, the first location, sometimes has the properties of six pulses, or it is lacking them, because of the approach and retreat of contrary pulses. Swimming and deep pulses are either short and long, or fast and thin, but those that are swimming come from primordial heat, and those that are deep come from radical wetness. So why did we say that these pulses from one source of wetness and one of heat are *xin kie*? Are they deep and fast, which are *yĕ iñ ch yâm*, from one source of wetness and two of heat; *Xim kie chaṁ*, deep, fast, and long? Each pulse that we called *yĕ iñ sañ caṁ*, coming from one source of wetness and three of heat, is *feu kie ulli cham xi yĕ xim*: they are swimming, fast, long, and afterwards, it is deep, surpassing the others.

The pulses that we called *yĕ yâm yĕ iñ*, coming from one source of heat, another of wetness, are *feu lli ci*; they are swimming and thin; those that we called *yĕ yâm Ch iñ* come from one source of heat and two of wetness; *chaṁ ch chaṁ ci*, at once long, deep, and thin. Those that we called *yĕ yâm san iñ* come from one source of heat and three of wetness; *Xin ci le tuon xi ien feu* are at one deep, thin, short, and afterwards it an overcoming and swimming pulse. Pulses very similar to the path of organs and intestines are seen, as well as the good or bad health of each one.

Commentary: Pulses from one source of wetness and one of heat are deep and fast. In the third location of the left hand, it indicates the connatural condition of the bladder and ureters. If the same pulse appears in the first location of the left hand, it is

Michal Boym

opposed to the heart and the small intestines (because water, or the bladder, whose pulse is natural, suffocates the first which holds sway over the heart).

A pulse coming from one source of wetness and two of heat (for instance, a deep, fast, and long pulse), if it appears in the third location of either the right or left hand (which location is subject to radical wetness), it is clear that wetness is overcome by primordial heat. The pulse coming from one source of wetness and three of heat (being swimming, fast, long, and then deep), if it appears in the third location (whether of the right or left hand), it is clear that radical wetness is smothered and dies in the middle of primordial heat. Likewise, a pulse coming from one source of heat and one of wetness (that is, swimming and thin), if it appears in the second location of the right hand, is a pulse opposed to the liver and gall bladder.

The pulse coming from one source of heat and two of wetness (being at once long, deep, and thin), if it is found in the first location of either the right or left hand (which location is controlled by *yâm*) indicates a depletion of blood and spirits, because radical wetness overwhelms heat. A pulse coming from one source of heat and three of wetness (that is, deep, thin, short, and after those, swimming), if it is found in the first location of either the right or left hand, it is clear that primordial heat is being killed and suffocated in the middle of radical wetness. Therefore, it is necessary to look into the assigned pulse-location for each of the twelve paths and sources, and to take pulses at four times—and moreover, to resolve the changes in the six pulses, and from them, the natural or preternatural condition of the human body.

## *Model for the aforementioned topics*

| *Xin*, a deep pulse coming from radical wetness | Here, inhalation enters the bladder and liver. Both are *Xin* pulses, deep; but a deep, soft, weak pulse indicates the bladder and ureters, because it is radical wetness within radical wetness; that is, a path within another path of the same nature. And so it follows for the rest. | Breath | | *Hu* exhalation | |
|---|---|---|---|---|---|
| | | *Hum kie*, the stomach, receiving food and its tastes, has a remiss but small pulse, because it indicates the condition of the stomach | | It leaves the lungs and heart. Both pulses are swimming pulses of *yâm*, heat; but a swimming, short, think pulse indicates a lung and the large intestines, for it is radical wetness in the middle of heat. | A swimming pulse comes from *yâm*, primordial heat. |
| | | *Chum chan hie*, deep, long, and fast, indicates *han tan*, the liver and gall bladder, because it is in *chum chi can*, primordial heat within radical wetness | But a solid pulse indicates *pi*, the spleen, for their condition is connatural (wetness within heat and vice versa[285]) | | A swimming pulse that is great and soon scattered indicates the heart and small intestines, for it is primordial heat within heat. |

Inhalation follows taking in of wetness.  Exhalation leaves with heat

---

[285] *contra*, literally, "on the other hand," "opposite." Very terse.

Michal Boym

First of all, I declare: The six points in the hands have six pulses, which indicate a connatural condition for the organs and the intestines connected to them. Indeed, in the first location *cun keu* of the left hand, the pulse of the paths of the heart and small intestines is *feu ta san*, floating, great, and one that is soon dispersed. It arises from pure and undiluted heat, so it is said to be from heat within heat. In the first location *cuñ keu* of the right hand, the pulse of the paths of the lungs and small intestines is *feu túm ci*, floating, short, and thin. Is source is primordial heat, in the middle of which is radical wetness.

Since both pulses are floating, they tend towards *yâm*, primordial heat, whose spirits are carried upwards. Thus, *hu*, expiration, leaves the heart and the lungs moving upwards. Then, pulses of this sort are assigned to the first location of both the right and left hand, because they are eminent and floating there, and almost higher, just like the organs themselves in the human body. They indicate their connatural condition. They seem to be in the first and higher location before the rest.

Again, in the second or middle location *quan* of the right hand, which indicates the paths of the liver (located below) and the gall bladder, the pulse is deep, intense, and long. Its source is radical wetness, in the middle of which is primordial heat.

Likewise in the third location *chě* of the left hand, because it indicates the path of the bladder (kidneys) and ureters (located lower down) is a deep, gentle, weak pulse; its source is pure and unmixed wetness; so it is said to be from wetness within wetness. The third location in the right hand (which indicates the condition of the gate of life and the third region of the body) has such a pulse; and when deep pulses are carried downward from *iñ*, radical wetness, then *hiě*, inhalation, which follows radical wetness, enters the liver, bladder (kidneys), and gate of life, where radical wetness resides.

Thus, both the second location in the right hand and the third location in the right and left hand has deep pulses, because even the organs and intestines, whose connatural condition they indicate, are located in the location of the lower region, that is, the lowest location of the human body—that is, the second and third location.

Then, it was necessary for a middle to be placed between *hú* and *hie*, exhalation and inhalation (meaning between *yâm* and *iñ*, wetness and heat—or rather, between floating and deep pulses, since they are extremely divergent); thus, of course, the pulse is middling, moderate, remiss. In the middle or second location of the left hand, which is called *quan*. This pulse, if it is remiss and small, indicates a connatural condition with the stomach. But if it is solid, it indicates likewise a connatural condition with the spleen. Its source is a shared equal between *yâm* and *iñ* (that is, radical wetness and primordial heat), for because the spleen and stomach are neither above nor below the other organs, but are in the middle, the pulses that indicate the condition of both were necessarily middling or modest pulses; that is, they are neither floating nor deep, and even the location where they are found is middling—that is, the second location *quan* in the right hand, where their pulses are perceptible. Clearly, <they exist> over the measure of time (that is, the delay in the middle of breathing) that comes between *hu ke* (exhalation and inhalation), if there are five pulses; and <they are> in the pulse-beats themselves, if there are four; because in the course of one breath, a healthy perosn should have no more than have and no fewer than four pulses, as we have said above.

It follows that the first location in each hand is subject to primordial heat; likewise, the third location is subject to radical wetness; but the middle location is subject to radical wetness and primordial heat equally. Thus, of the other connatural pulses that are found, some will come from heat (those are floating, fast, and long), while others will come from wetness (these are deep, thin, short). Moreover, a pulse in the first location of the right hand that is floating, short, and dull-and-thin,[286] comes from heat. Wetness being within it (that is, coming from one source of heat and two sources of wetness), they indicate the inherent

---

[286] *obtuso-rari*

condition of the lungs and large intestines, which are mastered by the cold of metals. Because fire will oppose cold, the heart will oppose the lungs, and the overflowing great pulse of the heart will oppose the floating and thin pulse of the path of the lungs. A pulse thus found in the first location of the right hand indicates that the metallic nature of the lungs is being destroyed by the fiery heart.

In the first location of the left hand, the pulse that is overflowing, great, and that is soon dispersed, comes from primordial heat and is in the middle of primordial heat; that is, it comes from the sources of primordial heat. It indicates the connatural condition of the heart and small intestines; but water is opposed to dry fire, and so the bladder (kidneys) is to the heart; and thus its deep, weak, and fast pulse is opposed to the great floating pulse of the heart. Therefore, the pulse found in a left-hand indicates that is comes from water; that is, fire (the heart) is extinguished by the bladder. In the third location of the left hand, pulses are deep and fast-and-sharp and weak, from radical wetness, in the middle of which is primordial heat—that is, it comes from two sources of radical wetness (seeing as they are deep and weak) and from one source of primordial heat (seeing as they are fast). They indicate a congenital condition with the bladder (kidneys) and ureters; sometimes, in the third location of the right hand, they indicate the condition of the gate of life and of the third region of the body (the nature of which is watery, although they also have fiery qualities). Yet dry earth is opposed to wet water, the spleen and stomach to the bladder and gate of life; thus, a remiss and idle pulse of the stomach-path, when found in the third location (whether in the right or left hand) indicates that water is being destroyed by earth—that is, the bladder or gate of life by the stomach. In the middle or second location of the left hand, the pulses are deep, long, and intense (like a taut string). They come from radical wetness, in the middle of which is primordial heat (seeing as they are deep and intense). They indicate a connatural condition with the liver, over which the woody or airy Element of the Chinese holds dominion. Metals, however, are opposed to the trees or wet air by their own dryness; and so the lungs are opposed to the liver, and their pulse in each <hand>, floating, short, and thin, is opposed to the deep, long, and intense pulse in the liver.

Thus, when found in the second location of the left hand, it indicates that the trees or cold air are being destroyed by Metals, and the liver by the lungs.

In the second or middle location of the right hand, remiss as well as languid pulses reside. They come from the mixing of heat and wetness, and they are in the middle between floating and deep, short and long, fast and slow or languid. They indicate a connatural condition with the spleen and stomach. Earth holds sway over the spleen and stomach, but the wetness and subtlety of trees or air is opposed to the dry earth. Thus, the liver is opposed to the stomach, and the deep, long, and fast pulses of the liver-path are opposed to the remiss, languid, and slow pulses of the stomach. Thus, when found in the second location of the right hand, they indicate that earth is being destroyed by trees or air, and the stomach by the liver. But if you have noticed well that connatural pulses originate from primordial heat and radical wetness (and these pulses appear in the six hand-points, with the source-paths being in the middle),[287] you will easily notice that the pulses that tend to creep in are contrary and preternatural. Likewise, wherever they go off course (either being deficient or surpassing) from connatural pulses; and thus, however the sources of the connatural pulses are influenced, they are diminished or cast off from their proper connatural condition and disposition. Do not neglect your knowledge of the diseases that destroy wellbeing and bring about Death, for wellbeing consists of moderation between primordial heat and radical wetness, which the pulses explain; diseases consider of change and variations in them, but death in the dissolution, or victory, or excess of either one, or the destruction of either one.

It follows second: Since pulse-locations have some floating pulses, some deep, Chinese Doctors note well that floating

---

[287] *mediantibus*, could also mean "cutting in half," (from the verb *medio*, meaning "to halve" or "to be in the middle")

pulses (which are carried upwards) have lightness; and deep pulses have heaviness. These things must also be noted well, and the location of any pulse must be explored carefully, just as they have either greater or lesser heaviness in it—if their delay or approach, even as it sneaks its ways in like a stranger or a guest (as the Chinese tend to say), should be connatural with the skin and flesh, or with the nerves, or with the bones; for this will make it plainly perceptible where the disease resides in that location (meaning, whether it is in the bones or the nerves only, or whether it is even in the blood or the surface of the flesh).

It follows third: Not only is it necessary, by the way, to take pulses in the assigned pulse-locations over the span of one breath, so long as that pulse moves four or five connatural beats over the course of one breath, so that that path and source (meaning, of the organs and intestines) had a good disposition; but it is also necessary for forty-five or fifty beats to be found in the same pulse-location over the course of eight or nine breaths. If those same pulses are found to be steadily unchanged over that period of time, it will mean that that path and source (meaning, of the organs and intestines) not are faring well themselves, but so are the other paths and sources from which they come, together with that path and source.

## CHAPTER SEVENTEEN

*Whether the pulses that are connatural with the twelve assigned paths and sources (likewise the spirits)[288] persist in the left- and right-hand location for a healthy person; or whether they experience their own changes over the course of the year, and what the motion and cause of the changes is.*

N ote first: The Chinese have a lunar year, which consists of 360 days. This number contains six times sixty days (and this cycle of theirs creates changes in the twelve hourly letters and the ten yearly <letters>).[289] So, because there are four seasons of the year (each of which take up three out of the twelve months, or almost ninety days), the Chinese have devised a fifth season, or change in the year.

Indeed, both spring and summer, fall and winter, have been assigned 72 days each, out of 90 days, or three months. But for the fifth season, they have given eighteen days (which run from 72 to 90 days), taken from each of the four seasons. So it happens that four times eighteen makes 72, and five times 72 makes three 360 days, which make up a Chinese lunar year, consisting of five seasons or yearly changes among them.

Note second that not only are the organs and their connected intestines subject to the five Elements, but also each season of the year. For that reason, the mastery that the five seasons have over the organs and intestines is rightly called mastery of the Elements; and the mastery that the Elements have is rightly termed the mastery of the five seasons. Thus, it is said that spring has mastery over the air and trees; that is, the liver, which has their nature. The summer has mastery over fire (the heart); autumn has power over metals (lungs); winter has power over water (the bladder, or kidneys) and finally, the yearly season

---

[288] *spiritus iidem*, literally, "the same spirits," and grammatically, it seems that it must be performing the same function as *pulsus connaturales* (the subject). Very terse, exact meaning unclear.

[289] Meaning unclear. *horariatum* by context seems to mean "hourly" or "pertaining to the hour," but it seems to be an invented word.

(which is the longest time—eighteen days— for any of four particular seasons[290]) has mastery over the earth—that is, the spleen and stomach.

Not only did they divide the times of the year into five seasons, which indicate five significant changes; but the rest of the time, they found and distinguished still other variations and changes, smaller or less notable. They say there are 24, and in the first twelve changes, *yâm*, primordial heat, grows and increases; but *iñ* is diminished by the twelve paths of the human body, and so even the pulses that originated in it change. But they knew that in another twelve changes, *iñ* (radical wetness) grows and *yâm* (heat) is diminished, and the pulses likewise change. But an especially noteworthy variation and distinction in the pulses occurs over the five seasons of the year, which tend to be observed with particular care.

Text: the codex says the following: The path and source of diminished primordial heat in the third part of the body sometimes produces a great pulse, sometimes a small one, sometimes a long one.

The path of pure heat and the source of the large intestines produces the pulse *feu ta ch ton*, floating, great, and short.

The path of great primordial heat and the source of the small intestines produces a pulse that is overflowing, great, and long.

The path of great radical wetness and the source of the lungs produces a pulse that is intense, great, and long.

The path of diminished radical wetness and the source of the heart produces a pulse that is intense, subtle, and small.

The path of defective wetness and the source of the liver produces a pulse that is deep, short, and swift.

---

[290] Literally, "which is the furthest time of the eighteen days of any from the four particular seasons."

Of these six pulses, some are connatural with a healthy man; others appear when illness comes, whichever paths of the aforementioned pulses have predominant pulses (such that their Spirits tend to hold sway over a decent number of days in the calculated months). Thus, during the winter solstice, the path of diminished heat predominates in a cycle of sixty days; but in the following cycle of sixty days, it is called the path of pure heat; afterwards, the path of diminished radical wetness holds sway, likewise in another cycle over the course of sixty days.

Thus, since mastery over any particular source and path lasts for sixty days, and six times sixty makes 360 days, it follows that masteries of various properties appear throughout the year in the six paths. Those masteries of the three paths and sources of primordial heat, as well as the time of the day when they exert their influence, are of the utmost importance.

Commentary: Various spirits of radical wetness and primordial heat appear particularly during the seasons of the year. The winter solstice has completely perfect *iñ kiĕ*, radical wetness, which produces primordial heat. The summer solstice has *yâm kiĕ*, completely perfect primordial heat, which produces radical wetness.

The sixty days of the first cycle follow, at which time the path of diminished heat begins to produce predominant spirits, which are still small, because the season is cold. Thus, pulses tends to enter rather than leave; for which reason, they are sometimes large, sometimes small, sometimes long or short, all mixed together. Thus, the first sixty-day cycle, beginning from the time of the winter solstice, falls at the eleventh or twelfth moon, and those pulses indicate the condition of the third great part of the body and the gate of life. The second cycle consists of another sixty days (which falls on the first, second, or third moon). At this time, the path of pure and bright heat golds sway in the second order; the Spirits that then thrive come solid, and the time of the year begins to grow clearer and brighter. The pulses are floating, great, and short. They indicate the paths of the liver and gall bladder.

A third cycle of sixty days comes next (which fall on the third, fourth, or fifth moon). The path of great heat holds mastery at that time and in the third order. The spirits for this time are many and great, the time itself being very hold. Thus, the pulses come overflowing, great, and long, indicating the condition of the small intestines and heart.

Afterwards, at the time of the summer solstice, in the fourth cycle of sixty days, the path of great primordial heat hold sway (this cycle falls on the fifth, sixth, or seventh moon) in the fourth order. The spirits are perfect, and primordial heat is most perfect, and it begins to produce radical heat and its spirits. The season is hot and wet, and so the pulses are forceful, great, and long. They indicate the lungs and the large intestines.

The fifth cycle of sixty days (it falls on the seventh, eighth, or ninth moon). The path of diminished radical wetness holds sway during this cycle in the fifth order. The spirits of primordial heat are diminished and recover; but the spirits of radical wetness increase. The time of the year itself is lukewarm, even rather cold, and thus its forceful, subtle, and small pulses indicate the ureters.

The sixth cycle of sixty days (it falls on the ninth or tenth moon). The path of radical wetness holds sway at this time. The spirits of radical wetness at this time are intense and perfect. The season itself is col (even icy) and rainy, and thus the pulses are deep, short, heavy, or weighty, and they indicate the bladder (kidneys).

The pulses that we have enumerated cannot be called equal and completely connatural with a healthy person, but neither can they be called contranatural, or belonging to an unhealthy person. Yet we have related them here that you might thus understand how the three path and sources of primordial heat practice their mastery in the course of a year, and how they cause the pulses in the human body.

It follows that spirits vary according to the variety in heat and wetness, and so on.

And these are the things that were sought to complete the Medical key, for the things that are pursued have long since been sent to Europe, and printed almost too hastily. Thus, we shall again take over in describing these things, which must without doubt be sent to the printer again for correction. Because mention is made so often in this Medical key of the organs and intestines, as well as of the paths that emanate from them, it seemed appropriate to include here images or drawings of each of the things that are contained in their books. They have no anatomy, unless you wish to call the drawing that is added here "anatomy." Thus, it is likely that everything cited from has a greater tradition.[291] In addition, they say that, even in the body of a dead person, there are many things that break apart and disperse which exist in a living person; and so, in Anatomy, there are still many things that could be elude even the most astute Physicians. But as it happens, for the person who is looking into each path's origins and endpoints (to which they say the pulses correspond), many things occur that seem to be contradictory. For instance, in the liver, for example, which they put on the right-hand side, the pulses should be taken in the left hand; and for the spleen, along with the stomach, they should be taken in the right hand, although they are located on the left. Additionally, the veins through which the paths of the ureters is said to end at the feet, and in the same way, the path of the third region of the body moves from the hands to the head, since this path seems rather to look to the highest region of the body. Accordingly, one may doubt whether the three pulses of each hand are distinct from one another and in such an order as they correspond to the order of the three regions of the human body. They indicate that the regions' health is proper or unwell. It can rightly be asked what they mean by 'bladder,' which they seem to represent by a drawing of the kidneys (are they subordinate? are they other glands?). I do not know, for they compare this organ (which the Author of the medical key calls the bladder) to two large red beans, called *lum teu*. They say that they connect immediately after the fourteenth spinal vertebra, on the back, towards the side of both sides. They are each two finger-

---

[291] Grammar unclear.

measures and three parts from the vertebra. They are directly under the stomach on both sides, and correspond directly to the navel. In the middle is the gate of life (primordial heat). It is situated between radical wetness, like between two gates. The aforementioned kidneys emanate from the vein of of the heart, and the lower path or vein descends towards the great mouth, then climbs to the marrow of the spine on the back, until it reaches the middle of the head, the location *sui hi*, called the sea of the marrows (or rather, of the brain). There are likewise many other such things that I will pass over here, each of which will seem rather unbelievable and laughable to Europeans, unless you perchance believe that so many Doctors have been unable to follow the mind of the Ancients, who yet boast tenaciously that they have practiced their art over the course of so many centuries, content merely with that Empirical or experiment-based science of theirs. In fact, they cannot provide a philosophical rationale for their things, and if they can take any light from Europe, they will certainly be delighted to learn it, and will gladly confess that they went wrong in many areas, as they admit with their Mathematics and Astrology—although it is quite old, the Fathers of their Civilization reformed it using our European sciences, with such great praise and benefit following thus from Christian law.

As for the drawings given below, it should be noted that they only remark on those paths, or locations of cavities (which they seek and distinguish from one another using their own terms), in the order for burning or branding, and for needle-points within the muscles,[292] which skill was in tremendous vogue in those ancient times (when they were ignorant of pains, and thus internal diseases, and thus believed that if they suffered any illness that it came from the outside), but which today they honestly admit that they no longer follow, it generally having fallen away over amid the tides of history, being almost buried. It has thus far not been possible to follow the drawings of the individual paths through all their twists and turns within the organs and intestines, nor should a person think that they exist

---

[292] *acuum punctionibus inter musculos*, talking about acupuncture.

anywhere inside China. Therefore, they have described only the beginning and end of each path in their drawings, leaving out the inner turnings (like alleyways or streams in the veins) through which each and every path in the organ and intestine ends and is separates from another organ's path, as can be seen in the description and model of circulation. Absolutely every book says the same thing about this circular. Even if it perhaps seems bizarre to the European, especially when they assign a measure of 810 *cham* (which contains 8,100 lesser cubits) to the whole circulation over twenty-four hours, unless we should say that each revolution occurs in individual fourths of an hour, or at least a single one at each half hour, and in any case 50 revolution within 24 hours, according to the circuit of the heavens over 50 homes, which Chinese books also state. But I, being ignorant of such matters, will gladly let it rest, leaving the Medical skill capacity that the Chinese have preserved over 40 centuries to the judgment and critique of the greatest experts.

Since the remaining Tables that follow the five that have just been recounted all still exist in the Most Noble Master Andreas Cleyer's *Specimen of Chinese Medicine* (Frankfurt, 1682), we do not wish to repeat them here. Rather, we direct the curious reader to that book; we shall only indicate the variation observed in the drawings. Meanwhile, the fifth table reveals a better method of taking pulses under <the wrist>.[293]

Table 5, which compares to Table I in Cleyer's treatise, has this inscription: A true likeness of an anatomically correct Chinese monster.[294]

Table 6 matches up with Cleyer's Table by number, as do all the rest; and to this sixth table is added this inscription: Image of the lung. The lung has a weight of three pounds and a similar number of ounces[295]; six leaves, two ears; it lies by the third joint of the spine on the back; it contains 24 cavities through which spirits are derived for the rest of the organs. The windpipe has

---

[293] *sub carpo*, exact meaning of *carpo* uncertain.
[294] Literally what it says.
[295] *uncia*, literally "a twelfth part," cognate to the word "ounce."

nine joints, or small rings. It is dilated during inhalation, contracted during exhalation. Note its path, and the path of the other organs and intestines, which it moves around in a circle. The lung begins fourth in order; it is completed ninth in order.

Table 7 comes with the following inscription: The path of the lungs, conveying great wetness, ends at the hands. It takes its beginning from the middle region of the body; that is, from the lungs themselves. It should be noted in these and the following drawings that only the middle part of the cavities is noted, for a determination must be made in that order also on the other part that corresponds to the same thing. It contains on the left and the right 22 cavity locations in total.

Table 8, with the following inscription: a drawing of the large intestines. The large intestine has a weight of two pounds and twelve ounces; it is two Chinese fathoms[296] and one cubit long (that is, eleven cubits), four finger-measures wide. But when it has circulation, it takes a measure of one *teŭ* of food, and seven and a half measures of water. Its upper mouth is the lower mouth of the slender intestines.

Table 9 has the following inscription: The path of bright head from the hands to the head for the large intestines; it contains forty cavity-location on both sides.

Table 10, with the following description: A drawing of the stomach. The stomach has a weight of two pounds and fourteen ounces; a length of two cubits and six finger-measures; it takes two measures of food and one and a half of water. Its lower mouth is the upper mouth of the slender intestines.

Table 11 has the following inscription: The path of bright heat from the head to the feet for the stomach. It contains ninety cavity-locations on both sides.

---

[296] *orgya*, a Latinization of ὀργυία, the distance of the outstretched arms (about 6 feet).

Table 12, with the following inscription: A drawing of the spleen. The spleen has a weight of 2 pounds and 3 ounces; it is five fingers-measures tall, three wide; the fat the sticks to it weighs half a pound. It is underneath the eleventh vertebra of the spine on the back.

Table 13, with the following inscription: The spleen's path of great wetness from the feed, ending at the heart. It contains 42 cavity-locations on each side.

Table 14, with the following inscription: A drawing of the heart. The heart is a pound, twelve ounces; it contains 7 cavities, 3 strands. It takes three small handfuls of purest fluid; it sticks to the fifth vertebra of the back. Four organs depend on the heart, under which they lie. The heart begins second in order; it is finished seventh in order.

Table 15, with the following inscription: The heart's path of the diminished wetness, from the heart itself to the hands. It contains 80 cavity-locations on both sides.

Table 16, with the following inscription: A drawing of the small (slender) intestines. Their upper mouth is the lower mouth of the stomach, and this is the upper mouth of the large intestine. They have a weight of 2 pounds 4 ounces, a length of 12 cubits. They have seventeen twists; they take nearly 2.5 measures of food and a little more than a measure of water.

Table 17. The same inscription is on this as is on the Cleyerian Table.

Table 18, with the following inscription: A drawing of the ureters. The upper mouth connects to the slender intestines. The weight of the ureters is nine ounces and two scruples.

Table 19. The inscription agrees with the Cleyerian table.

Table 20, with the following inscription: A drawing of the kidneys. The kidneys have a weight of one pound and two ounces, and they are fonts of water (seminal spirits), and thus of

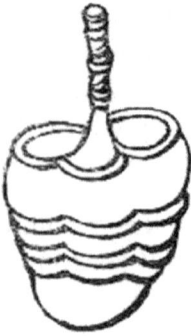

life and of the twelve paths. Within the afterbirth[297] (as they say) and within the smallest node of the navel, whatever arises there is the beginning of life; it is then divided on both sides into something like two shoots—or rather (as it seems) the kidneys.

Table 21. The inscriptions matches Cleyer's.

Table 22. It is not in the Cleyerian treatise, and it has the following inscription: the path of the pericardium, or the wrapper of the heart, conveying defective wetness from the chest to the hand. A drawing of it is given here, somewhat below the heart and above the diaphragm.

Table 23 is similar to the Cleyerian inscription.

Table 24, with the following inscription: A picture of the gall-bladder. The gall-bladder has a weight of three ounces and the same number of scruples. It has a length of three finger-measure, and it draws three handfuls of fluid.

Table 25. The same inscription as Cleyer's.

Table 26, with the following inscription: A drawing of the liver. The liver is located below the ninth vertebra of the spine on the back. it has a weight of two pounds and four ounces. On the right-hand side, it contains 4 leaves, but three on the left. It begins third in order; it is finished eighth in order.

Table 27, Table 28, and Table 29 agree with the Cleyerian tables.

---

[297] *secundinam*

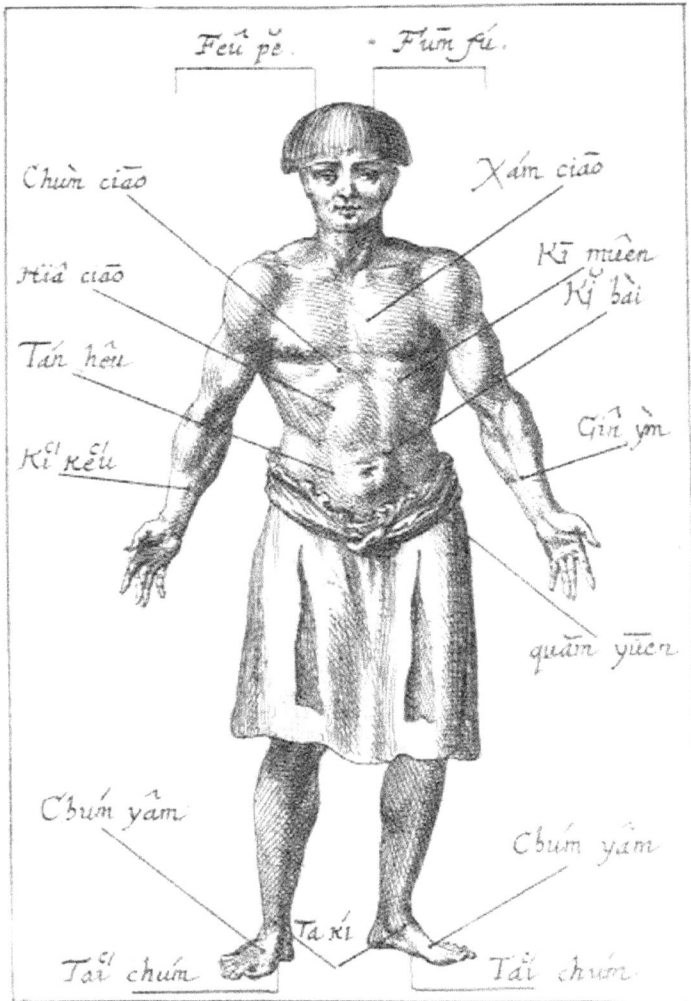

Feǔ pě.          · Fǔm fǔ.

Chùm ciāo          Xám ciāo

Hiǎ ciāo          Kī mùen
                  Kǐ bài

Tǎn hěu

                  Giǹ yǹ

Kǐ kěu

                  quǎm yǔen

Cbǔm yǎm          Cbǔm yǎm

          Ta kí
Tǎi chǔm          Tǎi chǔm

Ad Append. Annǐß

149

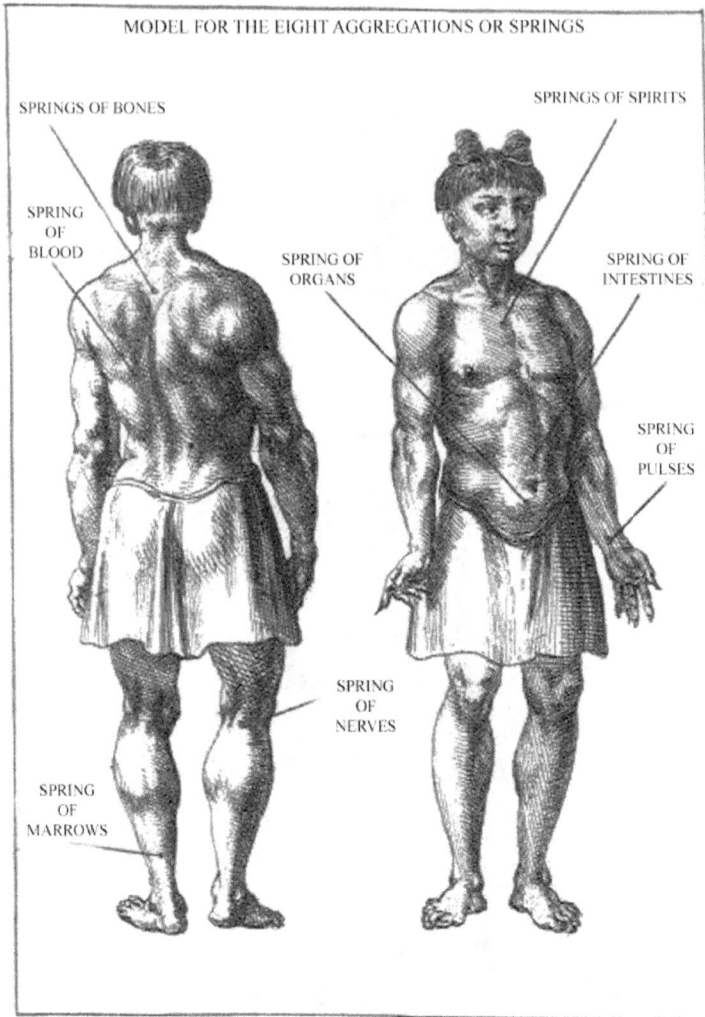

MODEL FOR THE EIGHT AGGREGATIONS OR SPRINGS

SPRINGS OF BONES

SPRINGS OF SPIRITS

SPRING
OF
BLOOD

SPRING OF
ORGANS

SPRING OF
INTESTINES

SPRING
OF
PULSES

SPRING
OF
NERVES

SPRING
OF
MARROWS

Dec.II.   fol.142

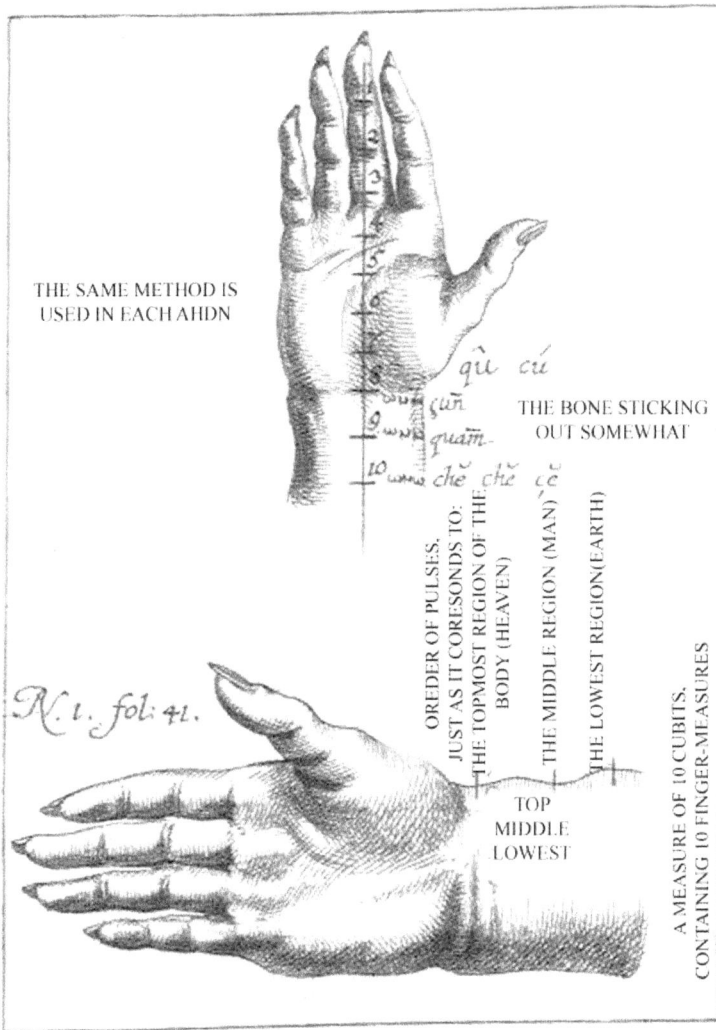

THE SAME METHOD IS
USED IN EACH AHDN

qù cú

çuñ

quãm

chĕ chĕ cĕ

THE BONE STICKING
OUT SOMEWHAT

ORDER OF PULSES,
JUST AS IT CORESONDS TO:
THE TOPMOST REGION OF THE BODY (HEAVEN)

THE MIDDLE REGION (MAN)

THE LOWEST REGION(EARTH)

A MEASURE OF 10 CUBITS,
CONTAINING 10 FINGER-MEASURES

TOP
MIDDLE
LOWEST

N. 1. fol: 41.

THE ANCIENT CODEX ASSIGNS TO THE FIRST LOCATION THE PULSE OF THE HEART AND PERICARDIUM. TO THE SECOND LOCATION, THE PULSE OF THE LIVER AND DIAPHRAGM. TO THE THIRD LOCATION, THE PULSE OF THE KIDNEYS (ON THE LEFT-HAND SIDE), AND THE SLENDER INTESTINES, AND THE URETERS.

THE ANCIENT CODEX ASSIGNS TO THE FIRST LOCATION IN THE RIGHT HAND THE PULSE OF THE LUNGS AND THE MIDDLE OF THE CHEST. TO THE SECOND LOCATION, THE PULSE OF THE STOMACH (BELLY) AND SPLEEN TO THE THIRD LOCATION, THE PULSE OF THE KIDNEYS (ON THE RIGHT-HAND SIDE) AND THE LARGE INTESTINES

THE FIRST LOCATION IN EACH HAND TENDS TOWARDS PRIMORDIAL HEAT AND CORRESPONDS TO THE UPPERMOST REGION OF THE BODY.

THE SECOND LOCATION SHARES EQUALLY IN HEAT AND WETNESS, AND CORRESPONDS TO THE MIDDLE REGION OF THE BODY.

THE THIRD LOCATION TENDS TOWARDS WETNESS, AND CORRESPONDS TO THE

ACCORDING TO MODERN TEXTS

ACCORDING TO MODERN TEXTS

*1* THE PULSE OF THE HEART AND SLENDER INTESTINES

*2* THE PULSE OF THE LIVER AND THE GALL BLADDER

*3* THE PULSE OF THE KIDNEYS AND URETERS

*1* THE PULSE OF THE LUNG AND SLENDER INTESTINES

*2* THE PULSE OF THE SPLEEN AND STOMACH

*3* THE PULSE OF THE GATE OF LIFE AND THE THIRD REGION OF THE BODY

THE ORDER OF THE PULSES IN THE LEFT AND RIGHT HAND, ACCORDING TO THE ANCIENT CODEX AND MODERN TEXTS, WHICH WERE AUTHORED BY VAM XO HO (FL. AROUND 1000 YEARS AGO). SINCE THEY TAUGHT (FOLLOWING THE CIRCULATION-ORDER FOUND IN THE ANCIENT TEXT) THAT THE SLENDER INTESTINES HAVE A STRONG ASSOCIATION WITH THE HEART AND WITH THE THICK <INTESTINES> WITH THE LUNG, THE JUDGED THAT THIS ORDER SHOULD BE SOMEWHAT CHANGED, ALTHOUGH MEDICAL AUTHORS OF THIS CENTURY CHALLENGE THEM. IT MUST ALSO BE NOTED HERE THAT THE KIDNEYS ARE DIVIDED INTO TWO SIDES, AS THE LEFT <KIDNEY> TENDS TOWARDS THE LEFT <HAND> AND THE RIGHT TOWARDS THE RIGHT, AND JUST AS THEY <SET THEM AT THE RIGHT HAND AND THE GATE OF LIFE, BETWEEN THEIRS AND THE KIDNEYS'>

*Tab. V.*

RULE FOR TAKING ONE'S OWN PULSE, BY EXTENDING THE RIGHT HAND AROUND TO THE PULSE OF THE LEFT HAND, SUCH THAT THE INDEX FINGER TAKES THE FIRST PULSE-LOCATION, AS BELOW.

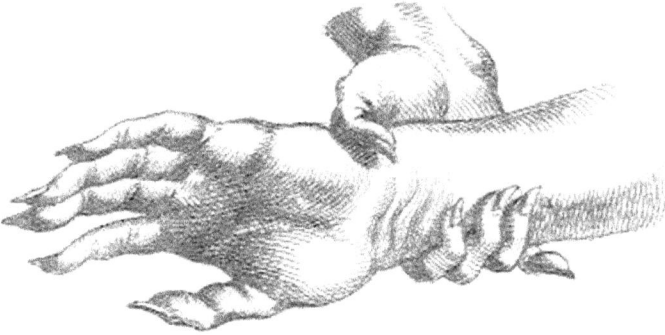

RULE FOR TAKING THE PULSE OF ANOTHER PERSON, SUCH THAT THE INDEX FINGER CORRESPONDS TO THE FIRST PULSE-LOCATION, THE MIDDLE TO THE SECOND, AND THE RING FINGER TO THE THIRD

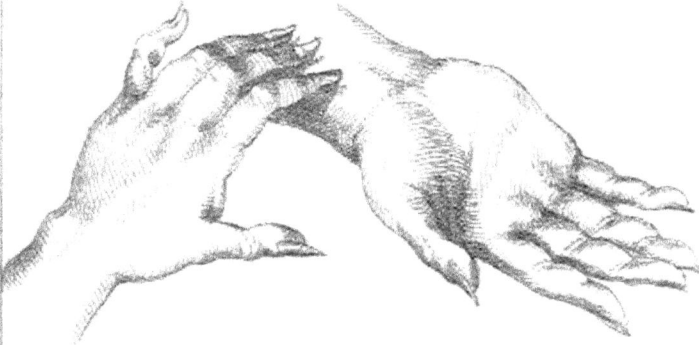

*N. Dec.II. fol. :42.*

Tab. VI.

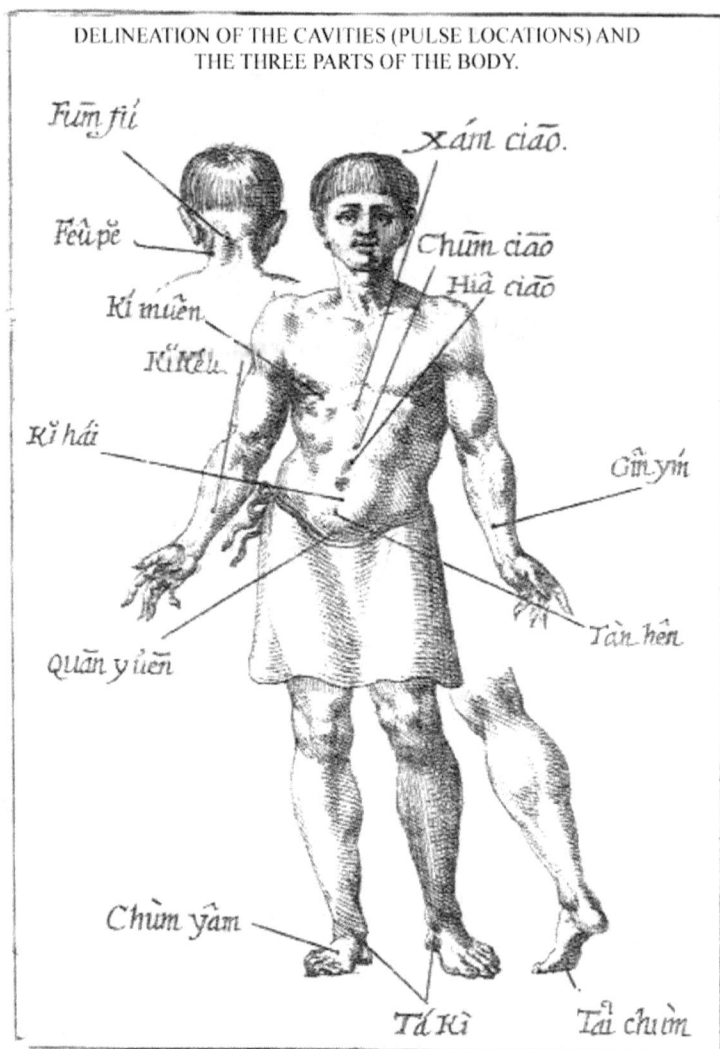

DELINEATION OF THE CAVITIES (PULSE LOCATIONS) AND
THE THREE PARTS OF THE BODY.

Fūm fíí

xám ciāo.

Feŭpĕ

Chūm ciāo

Kí muĕn

Hiǎ ciāo

Kî Kĕu

Kĭ hái

Gîn yín

Quǎn y ŭen

Tàn hĕn

Chùm yàm

Tǎ Kì

Tǎi chùm

Ad Append..

## Delineation of the cavities (pulse locations) and the three parts of the body.

**Fum fu**, that is, the city of winds. The location in the lowest part of the skull, where the furthest hairs indicate the condition of the lung.

**Feu pe,** that is, floating whiteness, a location in the back of the heat below the ears.

**Ki muen**, that is, the location of the extremities, below the breast; it reveals the source for the large intestine.

**Ki Keu**, that is, the mouth of spirits, in the right hand, behind the location *Quan*.

**Ki hai,** that is, the sea of spirits, a location one and a half fingers away from the navel.

**Quan yuen**, that is, the boundary of the sources, below the navel by 3.5 finger-joints. A vessel for perfect spirits. It reveals the source for the bladder.

**Chum yam,** that is, the penetration of the paths of primordial heat in the upper part of the feet, three finger-joints away lowest and furthest out <bone>. It reveals the source for the belly.

**Ta Ki**, that is, the great pond. These pulses at the sides of the feet, above the ankle. Men have them in the left food, women in the right foot.

**Xam ciao,** that is, the uppermost part of the body, from the top of the head to the topmost mouth of the stomach, below the heart and chest.

**Chum ciao,** that is, the middle part of the body, from the stomach to the middle of the belly. It contains the gall bladder, liver, stomach, and belly.

**Hia ciao,** that is, the lowest part of the body, from the lower mouth of the belly to the soles of the feet.

Michal Boym

**Gin ym**, that is, the course of a <meeting man>[298] (the paths of radical wetness and primordial heat). It reveals the source of the liver and gall bladder.

**Tan hen,** that is, the red field, a location three fingers below the navel.

**Tai chum,** that is, great penetration in the very center of the sole of the foot. It is called also the gate of life, because when the pulse stops here, a sick person dies.

---

[298] *obviantis*, see note on *obviatio*